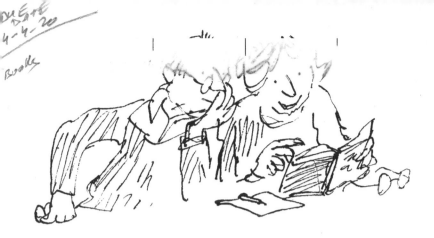

O ptimism helps you to live longer. *Feeling good!* is likely to give you a very positive view of life so reading it and following it could well contribute to your longevity.

Humour helps too and Alan Maryon Davis, whom I remember well for his humour, is a doctor who knows this. You'll find the book a very easy read, lightened many times a page by his deft, funny touch.

The book covers every aspect of your life and if you put only some of it into practice you'll be buying yourself many more active years of life. It's a wonderful combination: an MOT for later life and an instruction manual too.

One of the secrets of being as fit as you can be at any age is knowing that small changes make big differences. They're all in this book.

Dr Miriam Stoppard

Miriam Stoppard, well-known writer and broadcaster, is also the author of *Defying Age*.

Feeling good!

Published in 2007 by Age Concern Books

1268 London Road, London SW16 4ER, United Kingdom

ISBN: 978 0 86242 423 7

A catalogue record for this book is available from the British Library.

Edited by Janice Brown
Page and cover design by Kenneth Carroll
Reviewed by Margit Physant
Typeset by Intertype, London
Printed and bound in Great Britain by Bell & Bain Ltd, Glasgow

The publishers would like to say a special thank you to Martyn Partridge and Frances McInally of Intertype for all their hard work on this book.

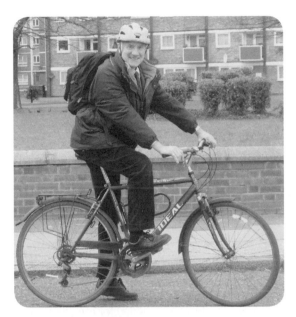

About the author

Alan Maryon Davis was a hospital doctor and general practitioner before specialising in preventing illness and promoting health. He is a prolific writer and broadcaster on health issues, familiar to many as presenter of the BBC TV series *Bodymatters* and *Save a Life;* guest on hundreds of radio programmes; and long-running resident doctor for the weekly magazine *Woman.* This is his tenth health book for the general reader.

In his spare time, Alan is an honorary professor of public health and chairman of the Royal Institute of Public Health. He enjoys walking, cycling, real ale, learning to sail and singing with the humorous group *Instant Sunshine.*

Acknowledgements

Warm thanks to: Steve Moore of Heyday for introducing me to the publishing arm of Age Concern; to Becky Senior, Commissioning Editor, for picking up the original rough idea and so expertly and patiently moulding it into something worthwhile; to Janice Brown for editing it into shape; and to my dear wife Anne for mowing the lawn, clearing the gutters, turning the compost, changing the plugs, putting up the shelves, and doing all the things I should have been doing while I was writing this book. I love her to bits and I promise to do the same for her one day.

Contents

Introduction

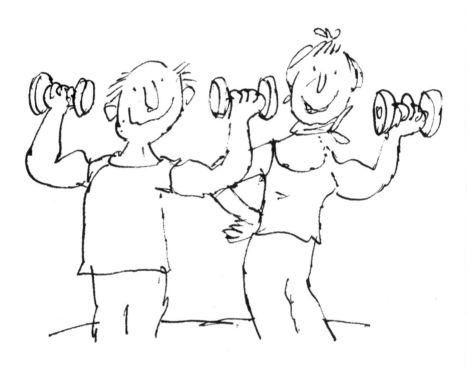

Do you feel that there's too much conflicting advice about healthy living these days? Or that it always seems to be more suitable for someone else and is never quite right for you? Perhaps you feel that the whole idea of healthy living is a bore – dreary diets, punishing exercise routines and very few pleasures. Or that it would be too difficult to fit into your life, taking up too much precious time. Or that it would just be something else to worry about.

Maybe you'd like to switch to a healthier way of life, but you think it's too late – like shutting the door after the horse has bolted. Or perhaps you find it far too complicated and daunting, and you can't quite see where to start.

Well, if any of these feelings ring true for you, then this little book could be just what you've been waiting for.

Unlike so many others, it starts with you – how you think and feel about your own health and lifestyle, and what differences you'd like to see. It helps you decide what to change and how to go about changing it. It's a simple, sensible, no-nonsense, practical and, above all, easy approach to improving your lifestyle and boosting your energy. It's about making the healthy choices the easy choices. It's about making life more enjoyable and fulfilling. And it's about taking things one step at a time, making small changes in ways that suit you at a pace that fits your daily life.

Small changes make a big difference.

Know
yourself

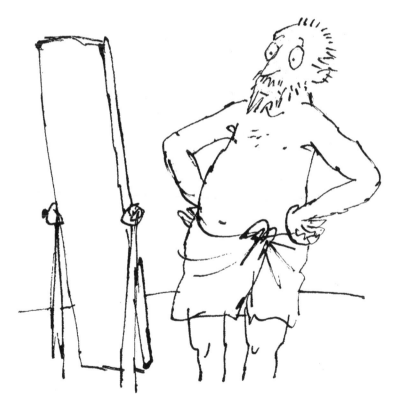

When you were young, 'health' was something older people worried about. You never gave it headspace. It was about as relevant to your life as yak droppings. Every day you would wake up, probably around lunchtime, assuming that your body would just carry on where it left off. You fed it junk, pickled it, kippered it, threw it around, hated it, ignored it, abused it, and generally treated it in a way that should have been reported to the RSPCA.

But now you've come to realise that not only is your body the only one you've got, but it's also at least a quarter of a century older than you would like it to be. Something has happened to it while you were having all that fun. Over the years it has tagged along, faithfully and more or less uncomplainingly, but now it's beginning to lose its sparkle and become a little frayed at the edges. And that's just the visible bits. Goodness knows what's going on inside.

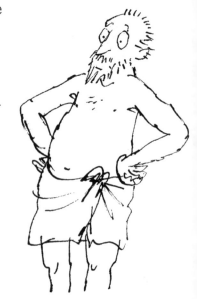

Fortunately there's still time to take matters in hand and do whatever can be done to reduce the ravages of time – perhaps even reverse some of them.

So, to get us started, here's a quick self-assessment fitness and well-being check.

20 questions to check your fitness and well-being

Here is just a quick run-through of some of the main factors that might have an impact on your health. The idea is simply to get you thinking and help you take stock. It might also be useful to revisit the questions in, say, 6 months' time to see if you've managed to make a difference.

1 Do any of the following apply to you?

- I wish I could lose a few inches off my tummy/hips/thighs/ other bit.
- I haven't got a fraction of the energy I used to have.
- I'm getting so stiff. I've got to do something about it.
- I'd like to give up smoking, but it's so hard.
- I haven't had a good night's sleep in ages.
- I know I drink too much, but so what?
- Relax? How can I relax when there's so much to do?
- I'm not quite sure what healthy eating is exactly.
- I'm tired all the time.
- Where did our love go?
- I feel all washed up.

IF YES, join the club. We've all been there. You can't really get to our age without having something threatening your health and well-being. And I'm so glad you're reading this book because you'll find it's crammed with good ideas to help you tackle some of these threats. Small changes really can make a big difference.

IF NO, I don't quite believe you. I did say if any of them apply, not all of them!

2 Do you quickly get short of breath walking upstairs or uphill?

IF YES, this is a clear sign not only that you're not as fit as you should be, but that you're probably nowhere near active enough. Physical inactivity increases the risk of high blood pressure, obesity, diabetes, heart trouble and a string of other problems. You really need to improve your stamina (staying power). The best way to start is by walking more, including more walking upstairs and uphill – something you can do straight away. But perhaps not just at the moment because we're doing this check-up.

IF NO, good to hear it. Let's see how you do with the other questions.

3 Do you struggle to get out of low armchairs?

If YES, you need to build up your strength – especially in your legs, but maybe also in your arms and trunk. The answer is to do some strengthening exercises such as those in the next chapter. The other answer is to buy higher armchairs.

If NO, more good news. Keep it up.

4 Do you find it difficult to bend down to tie your shoelaces or pick up things from the floor?

If YES, you need to improve your trunk suppleness by daily stretching exercises or some regular 'bendy' activity such as swimming, badminton, tennis or keep-fit. People often think that stiffness is an unavoidable part of getting older. But this is not so. It's usually simply due to your muscles shortening because they're not being stretched enough.

IF NO, you're not a ballet dancer by any chance, are you?

5 Do you find it difficult to reach awkward places on your body when you are doing up your bra-strap, for example, or combing your hair at the back?

If YES, you need to develop suppleness in your shoulders through activities or exercises that move your arms a lot. Again, badminton and swimming are particularly good for this. So is directing traffic.

If NO, maybe you're a traffic policeperson?

6 Can you put your big toe in your mouth?

IF YES, brilliant.

IF NO, I'm not surprised – neither can I. Only very keen yoga practitioners and contortionists can still do this in their middle years, although perhaps it's something we should all aspire to.

7 How much exercise or physical activity do you have in a typical week?

Hardly any (apart from very light everyday activity). You're in danger of seizing up completely. More important, your inactivity is risking depression, obesity, osteoporosis, high blood pressure, diabetes, heart disease, back trouble and a string of other disorders.

A fair amount (some regular moderate activity, such as brisk walking or fitness exercises, but not as much as the recommended amount – see below). You're doing really well, but not quite well enough. Build up the time you devote to moderate physical activity, sport or exercise. Even 10 minutes here and there will count towards your total.

Quite a lot (a total amounting to at least 30 minutes of moderate exercise on at least 5 days a week). Very good. This is the recommended minimum level for all-round good health and well-being. Make sure you keep it up, especially through the winter months.

8 Do you eat at least five portions of fruit or vegetables in a typical day?

IF YES, good, but why not aim for more? In some countries they're now going for nine a day.

IF NO, you're probably missing out on vital nutrients. See page 64 to find easy ways to make sure you take your five. Remember that a drink of fruit juice can count as one of your five, but potatoes can't.

9 Do you eat fish every week?

IF YES, the recommendation is twice a week and at least one of these portions should be oily fish such as sardines, salmon or mackerel, as these provide certain essential fatty acids which are good for the heart and circulation.

IF NO, maybe you're a vegetarian, in which case you can obtain the fatty acids through a plentiful intake of nuts and seeds.

10 Do you eat wholegrain cereals, wholemeal bread, wholegrain rice or wholewheat pasta on most days of the week?

If NO, it's best to have at least one portion on at least 4 days a week. Unrefined starchy foods should form the staple of your usual eating pattern.

11 Do you find it difficult to resist chocolates, crisps, biscuits and other wicked things?

IF YES, me too. But we do have to exercise some restraint don't we? See 'Eating well' for tips on how to wallow in a healthy diet and look and feel much better for it.

12 Do you drink more than the sensible daily or weekly limit for alcohol?

Go on – tot 'em up. How many lunchtime glasses of wine or pints of beer? And how about the evenings? More wine? A gin and tonic or two? A satisfying single malt? See page 128 to work out how many units that adds up to. Probably more than you think. The sensible limit recommended for women is not more than 2 or 3 units in 24 hours, or 14 units a week. For men, it's not more than 3 or 4 units in 24 hours, or 21 units a week. Remember that we tolerate alcohol less well as we get older.

If YES, you might have the beginnings of an alcohol problem.This won't necessarily show itself in obvious ways such as memory lapses or strained relationships, but you may be building up to a more serious problem such as high blood pressure or liver trouble. See page 123 for advice on how to enjoy drinking without tears.

13 Do you smoke cigarettes?

If YES, daily, you know the score. But check out the tips for giving up on page 119. There may be something that you haven't already tried.

If YES, occasionally, remember that there's no such thing as a safe cigarette. Every cigarette does some damage. My advice is to become a complete non-smoker.

If NO, but I used to – brilliant! Best thing you ever did for your health. You're reaping the rewards right now.

If NO, I've never been a smoker – even better. But if you spend significant amounts of time in a smoky atmosphere you may still be at risk.

14 Are you overweight?

Use this chart as a 'plumpometer'. Find your height (without shoes) on the vertical scale and run your finger across the chart until it reaches your weight (without clothes) on the horizontal scale. The shaded diagonal band gives your plumpness rating. Are you overweight, obese or severely obese?

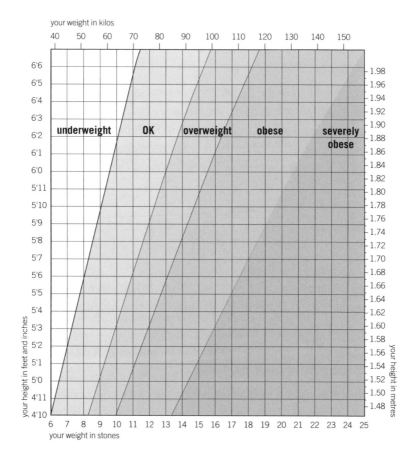

If YES, I'm sure you know what to do, but there are plenty of tips on how to lose weight and keep it off in this book.

15 Are you having all your regular check-ups?

If NO, you could be missing important opportunities to head off future health problems or nip them in the bud. See the 'Body check' chapter to find out what the main check-ups are for and where to find more information.

16 Do you usually sleep well?

If NO, this is likely to be affecting your health and well-being in all sorts of ways. 'Stressing less' suggests a few ideas for a better night's sleep.

17 Do you find it difficult to relax?

If YES, perhaps it's hardly surprising when there's so much to be done and to be concerned about. But there are ways in which you can use just a few spare minutes to achieve a state of deep relaxation. See page 115 for details.

18 Are you happy with your sex life?

If NO, why not? We look at some of the most common difficulties in 'Playing safe', and suggest some sources of help.

19 Do you quite often feel depressed?

If YES, you're in good company. Many of us feel downhearted more often in our middle years. We tend to worry more, often about things that younger people would shrug off as part of life's rich chaos. We may also feel low because of an 'empty nest', failing health or missed opportunities. Fortunately, even the bleakest of circumstances can be helped by taking a few simple steps. The last chapter in this book looks at ways of getting much more out of life – more engagement, contentment, happiness – in short, more *life* out of life.

20 In general (and not wishing to tempt Providence), would you say that, for your age, your health at the moment is good?

If NO, I'm so glad you're reading this book. You will almost certainly find there are quite a few things you can do to really make a difference and help yourself back to full health.

And even if your answer is a resounding **YES,** you will still find plenty of practical ways to hold onto your youthful vitality, vigour and well-being.

Small changes, big difference

I hope that this quick 20-question healthcheck has given you at least a taster of the aspects of your life you might need to work on. Rather a lot perhaps.

But don't panic. You don't have to climb the whole mountain, and certainly not all at once. Just take things a little at a time. A little change here, a small improvement there, gradually building more and more on what you've achieved. Every small step towards a healthier way of life is a giant leap for your well-being.

And talking of steps and leaps, let's kick off with the whole vital business of being more physical.

Being more active

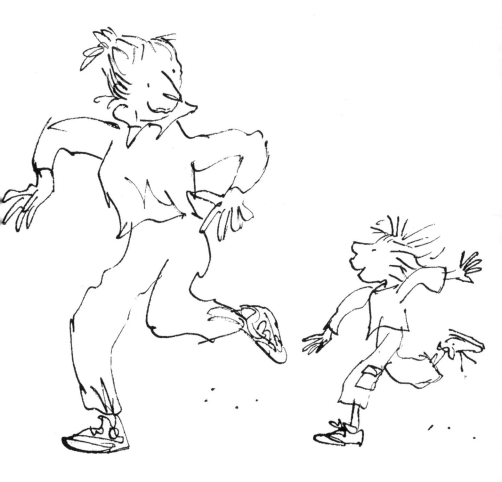

This is the big one – for your mind as well as your body. And, in many ways, this is the most important chapter of the book. Being more active could have the greatest impact on your quality of life.

Our health and well-being in the second half of life are partly determined by how well we've looked after ourselves in the first half. That, plus the set of genes we've been handed by our parents. Even so, there's still a great deal we can do right now to give our health a boost and to help us get the best out of life. Being more active plays an important part.

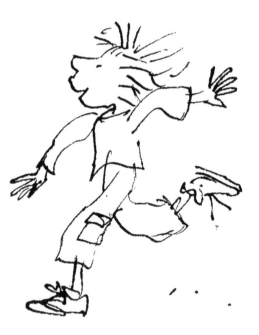

Excuses, excuses

Many people in later life think physical activity and exercise are not for them. They would rather watch other people doing it than take part themselves. People come up with all sorts of reasons for not being more active. Here are a few of the more predictable ones, and the counter-arguments for making a bit more effort.

It's too much like hard work

Who said anything about hard work? You just need to do a little more than you're used to, that's all. And by choosing activities you enjoy, and building up gently and gradually, it won't seem like hard work. As you get fitter, you'll find it easier and you'll enjoy it more.

I'm not the sporty type

You don't have to do sporty things to be more active. You don't need to don a leotard or trainers, or go to the gym or leisure centre. You just need to move around a bit more. If the word 'exercise' conjures up painful memories of dreaded school PE sessions, banish it from your mind. You can be more active without doing any 'exercise' at all. And you don't need to go anywhere near a PE teacher ever again.

I rush about too much as it is and need to relax

Nice try. But is your rushing about truly active – physically? Or are you in and out of the car, or turning from one task to another, without actually *moving* much?

Physical activity can be a great way to unwind and relax. Rhythmic dynamic exercise – like walking, running and swimming – can clear your mind and relieve stress, and afterwards you'll feel a lovely warm glow. Exercise can also improve the quality of your sleep and lift depression.

I simply haven't got the time to spare

This is a favourite. A kind of 'can't you see I'm busy?' brush-off. But it's based on the false idea that exercise needs to carve great chunks out of your hectic schedule.

Not so. There are all sorts of ways you can fit active alternatives into your everyday life. Being active needn't stop you doing other things. In fact, it can be energising. It can speed you up so that you're able to cram even more into your busy life.

I can't because of my bad back/knees/hip/heart/chest …

Exercise can be positively therapeutic for all these things and many more, so long as it's the right kind of exercise and you go about it in the right way. Your GP should be able to advise you on this.

The benefits

There's no getting away from it – exercise is good for us. The human body thrives on regular physical activity. And, just as clearly, a lack of activity adversely affects our health and well-being. Being more active can bring excellent returns.

Broadly speaking, the more active we are, the greater the benefits. The biggest gains tend to come when we move from couch potato to taking at least some regular exercise, and there are further benefits as we step up to becoming moderately active.

The people to blame are our Stone Age ancestors, who started this need to rush around. The earliest humans were hunter-gatherers who survived on a largely vegetarian diet of grains, roots, pulses and fruit, with meat or fish as an occasional treat if they got lucky with their spears. Their lives were quintessentially physical, and their bodies were built as lean machines to find food and water, build shelter and defend their families against attack.

It's only very recently in the timeline of human evolution that the amount of calories we take in through eating has exceeded those we burn up through physical activity. Thanks to the industrial revolution and, more recently, countless labour-saving devices from the motorcar to the electric toothbrush, we can now go through life without having to lift a finger. The consequence is a spate of chronic conditions such as obesity, heart disease and type 2 diabetes, which are all too often brought on by our inactive lifestyle.

> Did you know? People who make moderate exercise a regular part of their lives have about half the risk of dying from heart disease as inactive people of the same age, and they can also cut their risk of high blood pressure, type 2 diabetes and stroke.

Controls weight

A big consequence of our labour-saving lifestyle is the ever-growing problem of an overweight and obese population (see the chart on page 8). About one adult in four in the UK is clinically obese; as we enter middle age, this creeps up to one in three. We just have to look around us to see lots of roly-poly fifty-somethings – especially men. Perhaps there's one facing you in the mirror.

Nearly three-quarters of middle-aged men are either overweight or obese, and women aren't far behind. The UK has the highest levels of obesity in Europe and, if current trends continue, we'll be rivalling the USA as the planet's plumpest nation. Needless to say, much of the blame for this 'obesity epidemic' can be laid fairly and squarely at our own woefully inactive feet.

Strengthens bones and joints

One of the main benefits of active living is the boost exercise gives our bones and joints. From our late twenties onwards our bones begin to lose their mineral content and, along with that, some of their strength and durability. This is especially the case for women after the menopause, when the lack of oestrogen greatly accelerates mineral loss and increases the risk of osteoporosis, or so-called 'brittle bones' (see 'Body check').

> **Did you know?** Physical activity can help to prevent osteoporosis. It may also be beneficial for back pain and osteoarthritis.

The best types of activity to build up bone and joint strength are those that put some stress on the arms and legs – for example, jogging, skipping or tennis – but any activity in which you have to bear your own weight is good, even walking.

Activities like swimming and cycling, which don't involve bearing weight, are less effective for strengthening the bones and joints, although they can do wonders for muscle strength and stamina.

Promotes well-being

One of the real joys about being active is that it *gives* joy. As long as you go about it the right way, and stay within your comfort zone, it can lift your spirits and give you a real buzz.

There's plenty of scientific evidence to back up that feeling of a 'natural high'. Moderate exercise has been found to boost brain hormones called endorphins, which act as inbuilt antidepressants and tranquillisers. Rhythmic activities like running, skipping, walking and dancing can promote a feeling of well-being that lasts for some time after the activity stops. Sport and exercise are great for beating stress and reducing tension, and are often more effective at dealing with depression than popping lots of mind-numbing pills.

What exactly is fitness?

Funny word, 'fitness'. It's one of those words that means different things to different people. It conjures up images of sporty types, sweating away in the gym or pounding the paths in the park.

Feeling the benefits

There are encouragingly swift benefits from taking 'moderate exercise' as recommended by the Department of Health (30 minutes of moderately intensive activity a day on at least 5 days a week).

burning more calories	immediately
stronger pulse	almost immediately
greater alertness	within a few seconds
rosy glow	within a minute
toned muscles	a few minutes
cardio-respiratory adaptation ('second wind')	about 10 minutes
natural high	after one session
improved fitness	approximately a fortnight
stronger bones and joints	approximately 1 month
optimum fitness	approximately 6 weeks
lower blood pressure	approximately 2 months
reduced risk of heart disease	approximately 2 months

But being fit doesn't have to mean exercise machines, leotards and pushing yourself to the limit. It doesn't have to mean being able to leap about for hours without pausing for breath. For us over-fifties, with modest aims simply to feel well, have energy and get the most out of life, being fit means being able to do the things we want or need to do. Being strong enough to take the knocks and manage whatever lifting, shifting and carrying we may need to do without strain or injury. Being supple enough to reach those difficult places without a struggle. And having the stamina to run around with the children or grandchildren without collapsing in a breathless heap.

Your body has a remarkable ability to adapt to the demands made on it – even in your later years. It responds to activity by strengthening its working muscles, tendons, ligaments, bones and joints, by becoming more flexible, and by altering its chemistry to develop stamina or staying power. Providing you start gently and build up gradually over a period of weeks, your body will learn to cope and make the necessary changes so that the extra activity remains comfortably within your capacity.

Fitness is exactly this: it's the way your body adapts to demands, including the demands of everyday life. Older people may not be able to reach the level of physical activity or fitness achieved by younger people, but we can become *fairly* fit – and the gains we achieve in terms of capability, resilience, independence and health are well worth the effort.

Am I fit enough?

Good question. Something I ask myself every day. Not 'Am I tip-top, super-fit, the ultimate highly tuned human machine?' But 'Am I fit enough for everyday life? For the extra demands that happen from time to time? To help protect myself against such threats as high blood pressure, osteoporosis and heart disease?'

Fitness is not the same thing as health, although it's an important part of it. And being fit doesn't necessarily mean being healthy, although it certainly helps. Really, the most important question is: 'Am I *active* enough?' Perhaps we should leave the word 'fitness' to the sports coaches, exercise instructors and personal trainers. Let's just think in terms of how active we are and make an effort to move just that little bit more each day.

But if you want to, you can check your aerobic fitness with the simple step test in the box on the opposite page.

The three S-factors

Let's take a closer look at the three main aspects of fitness – strength, suppleness and stamina – sometimes called the 'S-factors'.

Step test

This is a simple home test of aerobic fitness. All you have to do is step on and off the *second* step of the stairs for 3 minutes at a pace that makes you no more than slightly breathless. Step up with one foot and follow it with the other. Then step down with one foot and follow it with the other – up, up, down, down. Hold onto the handrail if it helps.

After 3 minutes, stop, wait 30 seconds and measure your pulse rate. Count the number of beats in 15 seconds and multiply by 4 to calculate beats per minute. This is your 'recovery rate' – the measure of how soon your heartbeat settles down after exercise.

recovery rate for men (beats per minute)	recovery rate for women (beats per minute)	stamina level
under 90	under 100	very fit
90–99	100–109	quite fit
100–109	110–119	fair to middling
110–119	120–139	rather unfit
120 or over	140 or over	very unfit

Strength

This is the ability to exert force and is needed for gripping, pushing, pulling, lifting and shifting. We need strength all the time: to open stubborn jars, hold heavy kettles, move around, get out of chairs and carry shopping. Strength doesn't just come from strong muscles. Tendons, ligaments and bones also need to be strong. Strength helps to protect us from sprains and strains, and a strong back or trunk helps us to maintain good posture and avoid back trouble.

To build up strength, we need to use our muscles against resistance – to push or pull against something. In the gym, people use weights or machines; at home you can use your own body weight, for example by doing press-ups or sit-ups.

Suppleness

This is also known as flexibility: being able to bend, stretch, twist and turn, using our joints to their full range, reaching all those awkward places. We need suppleness for getting our clothes on and doing our hair, for getting in and out of the bath or car, for reaching for the bleach under the sink and doing all those fiddly jobs around the house. By keeping supple, we can manage these things more easily and we're also less likely to pull muscles or get stiff.

Suppleness is particularly important as we get older. If muscles are not stretched regularly, they stiffen and shorten, which limits the movement of our joints. This is much more likely in our later years. We often talk about our joints being a bit stiff but really it's our muscles not being stretched often enough.

 To be more supple we need to do exercises or activities that gently and gradually stretch our muscles while firming up the ligaments around our joints. See pages 46 and 47 for some easy stretching exercises.

Stamina

Stamina is staying power. It is also known as endurance or cardiovascular fitness – the capacity to keep going with any dynamic type of activity, whether walking, running, skipping, cycling, playing games, swimming, dancing or wheelchair wheeling. Without stamina, we soon get out of breath, our heart pounds, we have to slow down or stop for a rest, and our limbs feel like lead. Stamina is all about how efficiently our working muscles, bloodstream, heart and lungs can take on board oxygen and offload

Know your S-factors

Here's a very rough guide to the S-factor value of various activities to give an idea of how much they contribute to strength, suppleness and stamina. Needless to say, what you get out of any particular activity depends very much on how much effort you put in – a little extra can make a big difference.

activity	strength	suppleness	stamina
aerobics	★★	★★★	★★★
badminton	★★	★★★	★★
climbing stairs	★★★	★	★★★
cricket (fielding)	★★	★★	★
cycling (moderate)	★★	★	★★★
dancing (ballroom)	★	★★	★★
dancing (rock)	★	★★★	★★★
digging	★★★	★★	★★
football	★★★	★★★	★★★
golf	★	★★	★
hill walking	★★★	★	★★★
housework (light)	★	★★	★
lawn mowing (non-powered)	★★★	★	★★
pilates	★★	★★★	
running (jogging)	★★	★	★★★
squash	★★★	★★★	★★★
swimming (moderate)	★★★	★★★	★★★
tennis	★★	★★★	★★
walking (briskly)	★	★	★★
weeding	★	★★	
weight training	★★★	★	★
wheelchair racing	★★★	★★	★★★
yoga	★	★★★	

carbon dioxide. Regular exercise to improve stamina, particularly through its effects on the blood and circulation, can halve the risk of heart disease and greatly reduce the risk of a stroke.

 The best activities to improve stamina are any that make us feel a bit puffed, which is why they are sometimes referred to as 'aerobic'. But don't be put off by that word: walking briskly can be almost as good for building stamina as doing aerobics in the gym.

How much, how often?

The short answer is that it depends on what you're hoping to achieve. To feel a bit less stiff and more supple? To be less puffed going up stairs? To be able to walk further or faster? To be more fit for the activities you enjoy? To get more out of life? To boost your health?

According to the UK government's chief medical officer, to benefit our heart and circulation, we should be aiming to do at least 30 minutes of moderate intensity activity a day on at least 5 days a week. It doesn't all have to be in a single session – we can break it up into, say, 15 minutes brisk walking to the shops and 15 minutes walking back again, or even shorter bursts of 5 to 10 minutes doing various moderately active things.

What is meant by 'moderate' exercise?

In a nutshell, it means any activity that makes you breathe a little harder and your heart beat more strongly – enough for you to be aware of it. You might also feel warmer, go a bit red in the face and perhaps begin to perspire. But it's not so vigorous that you have trouble keeping it up. Moderately intensive activity can be continued comfortably for quite a while without rest. If you find you have to slow down or stop, it's vigorous rather than moderate and you're overdoing it.

Of course, what is moderate for you will be vigorous for

someone else and hardly exercise at all for another person. It depends on how fit you are. If you're not used to it, you might find that walking briskly is something you can't keep up for more than 2 or 3 minutes without struggling for breath.

The important principle is to let your body be your guide. You will increase your fitness by doing just a little more each week than you're used to – but only a little. If you're finding it uncomfortable, then you should ease up. And if it's at all painful, stop straight away.

If you can find the time to follow the advice of at least 30 minutes a day, on at least 5 days a week, all well and good. But many people find fitting this into their lives difficult. Some assume that, because they can't commit themselves to the full amount, there's no point in doing anything at all. But that's making a big mistake because every little bit of activity helps, as long as it doesn't cause discomfort.

What about the risks?

I know what you're thinking. This long list of potential benefits is all very well, but what about the risks associated with exercise, sport and a more active lifestyle? What about all those sprains and strains, pulled muscles, sore feet, aching knees, broken hips and heart attacks that wouldn't have happened if you'd only stayed in your armchair with your feet up and your eyes glued to the telly? Well the fact is that most of these risks can be reduced to a minimum by taking a few simple precautions.

Start gently

Don't rush into a fitness programme, or even your new more active lifestyle, as if your life depended on it (although in many ways it does). If you're not normally fairly active, or are pretty unfit, start very gently. Be just a little more active than usual for the first week or so. Walk just a little more. Bend and stretch. If you're taking up a sport or activity that you used to do years ago, regard yourself as a beginner – even if you were a bit of a star in your younger days.

Build up gradually

Each week gradually do a little more, but don't do anything that is painful or uncomfortable. The principle is to get just that little bit extra out of yourself while staying within your comfort zone.

Mix and match

You don't have to restrict yourself to just one activity or form of exercise. In fact, it's better to have a variety of activities to ensure all-round fitness. That way you'll develop all three S-factors. Try to combine an aerobic (cardiovascular) type of exercise with something more stretchy or strengthening. So, for example, you might want to take up walking and yoga, or dancing and pilates, or cycling and golf, or swimming and tennis. Or any combination you fancy. Indeed, why not go the whole hog and join a circus? Maybe not.

Wear the right gear

The right sort of footwear is paramount. It's also important to wear comfortable clothes that don't make you too hot or too cold, don't chafe your skin and, if necessary, keep out the rain.

Do it properly

By this I mean that it's important to get the necessary training or teaching from a properly qualified instructor or teacher, or from a reputable DVD or book. Why not join a class or club? Your library or leisure centre will have details, or you can usually find a class by searching on the internet.

And afterwards have a nice hot bath

This is the icing on the cake. This adds another layer of feelgood factor. This is the reward for all your efforts. So indulge, luxuriate and relax. You've earned it.

Getting started

Ready, steady, go! Well, er, no – wrong idea. Getting started isn't about sprinting out of the front door in your brand new trainers one bright crisp morning. Nor is it about kitting yourself out in glossy sportswear and signing up for a year's worth of exercise machines and spa treatments.

These things may suit some people – and might be right for you at some point – but they're not the ideal way to get started if you've been fairly inactive for the last few months, years or decades.

 Throwing yourself at an exercise programme, wham-bam, is nearly always a mistake. Build up slowly and steadily, over a period of weeks, so there's less risk of sprains and strains and generally overdoing it.

The chances are you'll be more likely to succeed in becoming more active, and keeping it going, if it results from a change of attitude. By that I mean the motivation has to come from within you, and not be something you force on yourself.

What's needed is a realisation that trying to do things the labour-saving way isn't necessarily best for well-being. The idea is to move more, not less. Don't curse because you've left your specs upstairs yet again – the more often you have to go up and down those stairs, the better. See it as an opportunity. Out of milk again? Great – a chance to walk or cycle to the shop. Power-mower broken down? Excellent reason to get a hand-mower and start pushing. Yes, I know this may sound like self-delusion, and that you may be thinking life's too short to be doing everything the slow way. But to stand any chance of succeeding in becoming more active, you have to change your mindset. You have to see the value in using your body more, moving more, being altogether more physical.

What to wear

The good news is that most activities don't require expensive clothes and equipment. Light, loose, comfy clothes in a natural fibre like cotton and shoes that can take the action while letting your feet 'breathe' may be all you need.

On hot, sunny days, you'll not only need to stay as cool as possible but, if you're outside, will need to protect exposed skin from the sun. Depending on the type of activity, a baseball cap or wide-brimmed hat will help to keep the sun off your head and out of your eyes. Liberal use of a high-factor sunscreen may also be sensible.

In poor light the crucial thing is to be visible, especially if you're walking, running or cycling near moving traffic, in remote country or over rough terrain. Bright, perhaps fluorescent, clothing will ensure that drivers or rescuers will see you.

In cold weather it's a good idea to wear a number of thin loose layers rather than a few thick ones, and peel them off as you get warmer. It's also important to stay dry – cold and wet are a potentially dangerous combination that can lead to hypothermia. For walking in cold weather that also threatens to rain, you will need a waterproof jacket and trousers that allow some ventilation so that you don't become sweaty after the first half mile. A good sports or outdoor shop will carry a wide range of waterproof, breathable clothing made of material such as Gore-Tex®.

The same goes for hill walking in any weather. Hills have a mind of their own when it comes to climate, and a cold wet cloud can appear from nowhere, as I discovered to my cost when rambling in the Austrian Alps one lovely summer's day many years ago, wearing nothing more than a shirt and shorts. Somewhere above the tree line the bright hot sun turned misty, then vanished in a sudden fog, and all I could see were a few rocks and edelweiss just in front of me. Eventually, guided by the sound of cow bells and the church clock, I managed to stagger back to my chalet, teeth chattering and legs like lumps of lead.

Now to footwear. For a dedicated walking session, you'll need comfortable, lace-up shoes or boots that let your feet breathe. Walking in the countryside, or over rough terrain, requires thick but flexible composite soles with a good grip, and waterproof uppers that allow some ventilation. It's also advisable to choose a size larger than your everyday footwear to allow for wearing thick walking socks and for slight swelling of your feet during a long trek.

For running and many other activities, including indoor games like badminton, the answer is trainers. If we believed all those slick commercials, we might be forgiven for thinking that it's hardly worth stepping out at all without a pair of air-cushioned, go-faster, ultra-zoom, mega-thrust trainers – or what we used to call plimsolls. But, unless you're a dedicated athlete going for gold, there's little point in forking out for expensive designer footwear just because it looks good. Having said that, it is certainly worth choosing your shoes with some care. Look for a good thick heel that will protect against the jarring impact of running or jumping on hard ground, a soft collar that won't chafe your ankles, a low heel-tab that doesn't dig into your Achilles tendon and, as ever, good ventilation.

Think too about your underclothes. Make sure that they're comfortable and supportive.

The serious walker's kit

lightweight waterproof jacket	gloves or mittens (winter)	chocolate or energy bars
stout walking boots	sunscreen (summer)	water bottle (summer)
extra socks	insect repellent (summer)	thermos with hot drink (winter)
fleece (winter)	sticking plasters for blisters	map
warm hat (winter)		compass
wide-brimmed hat (summer)		rucksack

The not-so-serious walker's kit

dog

Warming up and cooling down

For any kind of vigorous activity, it's best to spend about 5 minutes 'warming up' in order to tone up your muscles and make them less stiff and more efficient. Warming up should involve some form of gentle aerobic activity such as running or jumping on the spot and a few simple stretches. It will mean that your muscles will be less prone to injury and less likely to be pulled or strained, especially if you're about to launch yourself into any sport or activity involving sudden vigorous movements like aerobics, tennis, badminton and squash. Warming up is important however fit or unfit you are, but it's absolutely crucial if you haven't exercised for a while. See page 46 for some simple warm-up stretches.

Cooling down is a way of allowing your body to slowly adapt to the resting state and avoid muscle aches and stiffness. It's more or less a repeat of a warm-up – basically about 5 minutes of gentle aerobic exercise and stretches.

Do I need a check-up first?

Fair question, particularly if you have a medical condition that might be aggravated by exercise.

In fact most people, even older people, don't need a medical examination before becoming a little more active. As long as you keep to the golden rules of taking things very gently and gradually, and never doing anything that causes discomfort, you shouldn't have any medical problems as a result of exercising. Indeed, all the evidence points to a long list of benefits.

But if you have a chronic condition such as high blood pressure, diabetes, a bad chest or arthritis, it is probably advisable to see your doctor or practice nurse beforehand, if only to find out whether taking up exercise might have an effect on any treatment you're undergoing.

Most of these long-term conditions, and a string of others, are improved by participating in appropriate forms of activity, and you might find that your doctor can advise you on which activities are appropriate for you. For example, if you have high blood pressure, it would be sensible to avoid activities involving a lot of straining against resistance, such as working weights or rowing. Instead, go for free-flowing rhythmic forms of exercise like walking, cycling or swimming. If you have arthritis in your knees, you may find walking uncomfortable, in which case, try a non-weight-bearing activity such as cycling or swimming.

Choosing activities

Needless to say, the choice is potentially enormous. There are so many active things to do – so many pleasant walks, leisure centres, sports clubs, dance clubs, health clubs and gyms – that it's hard to know where to begin. But here are a few basic questions to ask yourself:

❖ Do I want simply to be more active in my everyday life, or do I want to take up some form of leisure activity in a more dedicated way? You could do both of course.

❖ If the latter, what would I enjoy doing? Enjoyment is crucial, otherwise you're unlikely to keep it up.

❖ Would I prefer doing something on my own, or with other people? If with other people, would I like to join a club or team?

❖ Would I prefer doing an activity as and when I feel like it or on a more regular basis?

❖ Should it be something indoors or out? Bear in mind that it's just as important to keep active in the autumn and winter months as it is in the spring and summer.

❖ Can I be bothered with the special clothing, kit, training, etc that might be needed?

❖ Is it reasonably convenient? Can I get to it easily? Can I afford it?

❖ What's a good combination of activities to develop my strength, suppleness and stamina?

Being active has another great advantage: it can be an enjoyable way to spend time with someone. If there's a friend you don't manage to see very often, you could arrange to attend a regular exercise class or go swimming together. And a short daily walk can be a great way for busy couples to unwind together – and to remember what you like so much about each other's company!

Walking

This is a wonderful activity for people in their middle years, especially if you haven't been used to exercise for some time. It's easy, gentle, convenient, free and, if you want it to be, sociable. It's aerobic, so it's beneficial for your heart and circulation. It builds up the strength of your muscles, bones and joints. It also has the advantage of getting you from A to B, so you can use it in your everyday life.

Getting started

It's a good idea to start simply by walking as a way of getting about. Perhaps to the local shops or as part of your journey to and from work? Perhaps to visit friends nearby, or to take a turn around your local park? If you can take longer walks, you'll soon feel the benefits: easier breathing, stronger legs, a slimmer waistline and real relaxation. For me, one of the great joys of walking is getting away from the hurly-burly of the city, hearing the sound of birds singing and leaves rustling. Wonderful! Especially in my favourite part of the country – the Yorkshire Dales.

Try this 8-week walking programme

If you'd like to set yourself a regular programme to build up your walking fitness, here's a simple programme spread over 8 weeks.

weeks 1 and 2

Just find every opportunity to do a little more walking in your everyday life, literally every day. Use the stairs rather than the lift or escalator. Get off the bus a stop or two earlier. Walk your grandchildren to school. Walk the dog off its little feet. Do even more walking at weekends.

weeks 3 and 4

Begin the scheduled walking programme proper. Two walks each day of at least 10 minutes each without stopping. Try a longer walk of at least 20 minutes on at least one of your weekend days – strolling pace. Take friends or family.

weeks 5 and 6

Two walks each day of at least 15 minutes without stopping. Again, try a longer walk of at least half an hour on at least one of your weekend days. But build up the pace in the second week.

weeks 7 and 8

Now you should be aiming for a single daily walk of at least 30 minutes at a brisk pace without stopping. An hour's brisk walk on one of your weekend days would be excellent. If you manage 30 minutes brisk walking on at least 5 days a week you will be achieving the Department of Health's recommended level for optimum health. So keep it up – and enjoy your new vitality.

Led walks In most places in the UK you can join an organised walk led by a trained walk leader. These walks may be organised by the local council, health service or walking club. They may take place in the country, or in the town or village where you live. You can usually find a group through the local library or visitor information centre. There are often two walk leaders for each walk – one at the front of the group and the other at the back to keep an eye on stragglers. The rearguard can also provide a helping hand for anyone who has recently been unwell or is not sure how far they can walk.

Rambling If you want to go a bit further afield then there are a few basic rules:

- Choose clothing to suit the weather and terrain.
- Wear lots of thin layers to keep warm, rather than a few thick ones.
- Take a good map and your mobile phone, and tell someone where you're going.
- Take a drink and a snack.

 Two useful organisations that provide information on walking and led walks are: The Ramblers Association (telephone 020 7339 8500; www.ramblers.org.uk); and Walking the Way to Health (telephone 01242 533258; www. whi.org.uk).

Jogging and running

Ready to break into a jog? By stepping up a gear to this more vigorous form of exercise, you can achieve a higher level of aerobic fitness than by brisk walking (although stair and hill walking are more or less equivalent to jogging on the flat in terms of building stamina). Jogging is an easy-going form of running at a comfortable pace, while running can be anything up to Olympic Gold. But, for our purposes, there's really very little distinction between the two terms. 'Running' just sounds a little more cool.

The step-change for people in later life is that, unlike walking, both jogging and running involve 'high impact' with the ground. For most people this jarring effect is a good thing because it stimulates the bones and joints to become stronger and tougher, and helps to counteract the effects of osteoporosis (brittle bones).

Jogging and running are excellent for building stamina and burning calories and, as with all aerobic forms of exercise, will help to improve the circulation and protect the heart. But there's no real benefit for the upper body and arms unless you run with weights, which many keen types do.

There are, however, risks to running: pulled muscles, sore tendons, twisted ankles, twingeing knees, slips and trips. But these can be reduced by wearing good shock-absorbent running shoes and running on level and well-maintained paths. Believe it or not, one of the most common running injuries is a sprained or broken wrist, caused by slipping or tripping and landing awkwardly on an outstretched hand. Another problem, mostly suffered by male fun runners, is 'joggers' nipple' – soreness due to chafing by a loose T-shirt. Worse in cold weather I'm told.

It's probably best to avoid this form of exercise if you have arthritis or back trouble or are very overweight. Consider a low-impact activity that doesn't put stress on your joints, like walking, cycling or swimming, instead.

Getting started

The easiest way to start is to work up to it over several weeks, perhaps with a friend, solving the problems of the world as you jog along. Jogging in the park or along country lanes can be sheer pleasure, and the scenery changes constantly. Why not combine it with a nature walk? Frequent short stops are allowed while you inspect the odd toadstool, rare orchid or red squirrel. (I'm kidding.)

You will need different gear for running – comfortable thick-heeled trainers, perhaps a cap for a sensitive head, light,

Try this 6-week running programme

If you're ready for some running, try this simple build-up programme. The principle is the same as for walking: always stay within your comfort zone and always start and finish with a couple of minutes of warming up and cooling down (see pages 46 to 48).

week 1

Walk briskly for 4 minutes, then jog for 30 seconds. Alternate like this for as long as you can, but ideally 20 to 30 minutes. Try to do three sessions during the first week.

week 2

In the second week, walk briskly for 4 minutes and jog for 1 minute, repeating the pattern until you've exercised for 20 to 30 minutes. Do this three times during the week.

weeks 3 and 4

Walk briskly for 2 minutes, then jog for 3 minutes. Repeat for the rest of the 20 to 30 minutes. Do this three times a week for 2 weeks.

week 5

Walk briskly for 1 minute and jog for 4, repeating for the rest of the session.

week 6

In the last week, gradually drop the walking altogether, so that you're finally jogging for the full 20 to 30 minutes. From this point, you should try to keep your running going for as long as possible during each session, ideally at least three times a week.

breathable clothes, including shorts, and a long-sleeved top you can take off and wrap around your waist when you get warm. In low light, something bright or reflective is a must if there's traffic about.

Like walking, you can jog all year round, but it's best to avoid really wet days and icy conditions. And don't volunteer as a lightning conductor during thunderstorms.

 Two very useful websites for runners at all levels: www.runnersweb.co.uk and www.runnersworld.co.uk

Cycling

Apart from walking, which I love, this is my favourite form of exercise, and I do at least two half-hour trips a day, 5 days a week, to and from work in the inner city. It's not only good exercise, but also fast, silent, clean, convenient, purposeful, free and kind to the planet. Think of all the carbon emissions we could save.

Cycling is not an all-round form of exercise. It doesn't work equally for all the S-factors. It's fine for building stamina and burning calories, as long as you push reasonably hard (with hills to negotiate, you will have to), and it's good for strengthening the extensor leg muscles. But, because it's non-weight-bearing, it does very little to strengthen the bones and is pretty useless for the arms and upper body. If it's all-round fitness you're after, you'll need to combine cycling with other forms of exercise.

There are risks of course. Cycling anywhere other than in a dedicated bike lane requires constant vigilance. You need eyes in the back of your head to watch out for cars, lorries and motorbikes coming too close. And you need to be very careful turning right in fast-moving traffic. Bus queues can be hazardous too – on one occasion I was nearly knocked off my bike by someone frantically hailing the bus behind me.

A good helmet is essential. So are front and rear lights in dark conditions – I prefer the flashing LED-type – as well as a light-coloured or reflective jacket. Other essentials include a tough lock, rainproof jacket and trousers, and, for longer trips, a pump. I put all this stuff in a backpack – but you might prefer to put it, along with your shopping and other bits and pieces, in panniers or a basket on the handlebars.

Getting started

A good way to get started is to do short trips down quiet roads or cycle tracks at weekends or in the middle of the day when traffic is a little lighter. If you go with a friend, cycle in single file rather than side by side.

Look drivers straight in the eye when pulling out or crossing a stream of traffic. Always cycle confidently and take up plenty of space. Don't shrink to the side of the road.

If you haven't cycled for some time, another useful idea is to go on a short adult cycle training course. A nationwide scheme is run by the CTC, the national cycling organisation.

Information on cycling is available from the UK's national cyclists' organisation, the CTC, which has over 70,000 members and affiliates of all ages and abilities (telephone 0870 873 0060; www.ctc.org.uk). Contact the National Cycle Training Helpline (0870 607 0415) for information about any aspect of cycle training.

Swimming

Any kind of swimming is good for us – even pottering about at the shallow end or a quick dip in the briny on our summer hols. There's something about floating semi-naked in water that's a real tonic. OK, we may no longer have the body beautiful, or even bearable, but we shouldn't let such a trifling consideration deny us the pleasures of swimming. Unless, of course, we hate the whole business of getting changed, getting wet, getting dry and getting changed again.

Swimming is one of the best ways to stay supple while building and maintaining strength and stamina. It exercises all parts of the body – arms, legs, trunk – and if you use a variety of strokes you can quickly develop aerobic fitness and burn up the calories.

However, like cycling, it's non-weight-bearing (the water is supporting your weight) and therefore not as effective as walking or jogging for strengthening the bones in your legs and back. But it's very good for your arms and shoulders and all your joints. If you suffer from back pain or arthritis, swimming is truly therapeutic, helping to loosen you up and ease your aches. Indeed, many hospitals have hydrotherapy pools for just this purpose. It's also brilliant for people who are overweight. And, of course, swimming is wonderfully relaxing – a great way to soothe away stress.

Getting started

A good way to dip your toe in the water is to go along to your local pool, perhaps with a friend, at one of the quiet times. Or perhaps join an aquafit or aqua-aerobics class. Many pools have special sessions for the over-fifties, and if you can't swim, there are always lessons at concessionary prices. The only snags are that you have to undress and get wet.

 For further information on all aspects of swimming, contact British Swimming (0871 200 0928; www.britishswimming.com).

Aerobics and keep-fit

These are exercises usually done to music as a group in an aerobics class, or at home to a video or DVD. In most communities there are aerobics classes specially tailored to the older person, which means that the tempo is a little less frenetic and the exercises a little more civilised. The emphasis tends to be more on stretching than calorie-burning, and the movements are 'low impact', which means that they're kinder to the back, knees and ankles.

Aerobics and keep-fit classes come in various guises (such as dancersize, stretchersize, tums 'n' bums, trim 'n' tone) and they have two big pluses: one is that they are led by someone who is properly trained in exercising sensibly and safely (or they should be); the other is that, being a group thing, they're sociable – you get to know people, you bond with them and you keep going to the classes.

Getting started

Check out your local leisure centre or community centre to see what types of exercise class are offered for the over-fifties. There will usually be something that will suit you rather well. And if being sweaty in public is not your idea of a good time, then there are countless exercise videos and DVDs available, so you can have a go in the privacy of your own home.

 To find a keep fit or aerobics class near you, contact the Keep Fit Association (telephone 020 8692 9566; www.keepfit.org.uk).

Tennis

Tennis used to be a summer-only sport but with our increasingly mild winters the courts now tend to be open all year round. This is good news for us oldies because it means we can get out there and play a few sets before the young ones have even begun to stir from their beds.

Tennis is great for suppleness and stamina – lots of stretching and dashing about. It does of course require people to be in reasonable physical shape (no favours for a bad back or dodgy knee, for instance). But it's great fun, especially doubles, and you can play as artlessly as you wish, as long as your companions are prepared to put up with you. If not, you can offer to pick up the balls and pour the lime juice cordial.

Getting started

Who's for tennis? Why not find a friend who would like to try a knockabout and book yourselves into the local courts? Borrow the racquets and balls if necessary. What about a game of doubles, if you can remember roughly how to do it. Great fun. Or, if you've never played before, or haven't held a racquet in years, arrange for some private lessons with a local coach.

And don't worry about appearing on court in gleaming tennis whites. As long as you're comfortable, have a racket, a few balls and a pair of trainers, you're all set.

 For information on tennis clubs, events and tournaments catering for 'veterans' (anyone over 35), contact the Lawn Tennis Association (telephone 020 8487 7000; www.lta.org.uk).

Golf

There's something about golf that really takes people over. Perhaps it's the appeal of the great outdoors. Maybe it's the combination of gentle exercise, skill and competition. Or could it be the beauty of the fairways and greens? For whatever reason, golf is one of the most popular sports for the over-fifties, and our clubs and municipal courses are thronging with people like us having a wonderful time whacking a little white ball around a stretch of rolling countryside.

On top of all that, it's healthy too. Walking for 18 or even 9 holes helps to build up stamina. Practising your swing keeps you supple. And the companionship and open air are good for the soul. All in all, it's well worth taking up and needn't cost a fortune if you play the municipal courses.

Getting started

A good place to start is your local putting green. A few sessions will remind you how the putter and ball need to work together, and force you to concentrate on grip and stance.

Then you'll need to move up to the big stuff – driving. As well as grip and stance, the thing to master is the swing. You can practise this most easily at one of those special driving ranges, where you can usually also hire some tuition. You could also buy a book on the basic techniques.

Soon you'll be able to graduate to the real thing – the 9-hole and then the 18-hole course, either on your own or with a partner. Most courses will rent you a basic set of clubs.

For golfing beginners in England, a good starting point is the Get into Golf website (www.getintogolf.org). In Scotland, the official body is the Scottish Golf Union (telephone 01382 549500; www.scottishgolfunion.org). The National Association of Public Golf Courses can provide details of inexpensive golf courses (telephone 01527 542106; www. napgc.org.uk).

Bowls

This is another very popular activity for older people, although it's catching on with many younger players too. Bowls comes in a number of varieties, from lawn bowls to ten-pin, and from crown green bowls to short-mat. But the classic picture of bowls in your local park is a group of older people dressed in white cotton skirts or trousers and dark blue blazers, skilfully launching their heavy lignum bowls in subtle arcs across the manicured green.

Getting started

Apart from the bending and stretching, the exercise value is minimal. You really won't have to worry about what level of fitness you're at, as long as you can swing an arm and pick things up from the floor. The real value of bowls lies in its social value – bowls players often build up friendships that endure for decades – as well as its tendency to take your mind off things. So why not get a few friends together for a special occasion and give it a shot?

For further information on bowling, contact the
English Bowling Association (www.bowlsengland.com),
the Scottish Bowling Association (www-scottish-bowling.
co.uk), the Northern Ireland Bowling Association
(www.nibabowls.co.uk) or the Welsh Bowling Association
(www.welshbowlingassociation.co.uk).

Dance

Whether your thing is rock 'n' roll, jive, ballroom, salsa, tap, line-
dancing, lindy hop, ballet or any of the countless forms of traditional
dance, moving to music is one of life's special pleasures. As an
expression of togetherness, celebration and sheer good fun,
dancing is enjoyed by cultures throughout the world. It can also be
very healthy exercise. Depending on the type of dancing and how
energetic it is, it can be good for suppleness, strength and stamina.
Dancing offers something for everyone. Even if you're the clod-
hopping, bulldozer type with two left feet and no sense of rhythm,
you can still enjoy jumping up and down without doing too much
damage to those around you.

Getting started

Most communities, adult education centres, leisure centres and
clubs have regular sessions for various forms of dance. Although
it's certainly easier to go along with a friend or partner, dance events
tend to be good ways to meet people in your local area. If you don't
want to commit to a full course, you can often opt for a one-off
taster session. If there's nothing locally, perhaps you and some
friends could get something started by contacting the Foundation
for Community Dance (see page 42).

Keep an eye open for the adverts in your local paper or library,
check the council website and get out your little sequinned number
or that slightly off-white tuxedo. Let's boogie!

Further details and news on dance events are available from the Foundation for Community Dance, a UK-wide charity working to bring the benefits of dance to communities and individuals (www.communitydance.org.uk).

Pilates

Pilates is an approach to exercise that focuses mainly on the core set of muscles in the trunk and back and involves the principles of control, concentration, positioning, posture, fluidity and breathing. But it's also a philosophy – a way of going through life being aware of the position, balance and movement of your body.

Pilates is a very gentle way of exercising that's particularly useful for people with back problems who might have trouble with other forms of exercise.It is also often appropriate for people recovering from physical injury.

However, while pilates develops strength and suppleness, it doesn't involve aerobic exercise and won't significantly improve stamina or cardiovascular health.

Getting started

It's best to join a class led by a properly qualified pilates instructor (to at least Level 3). Beware those who have not received adequate training. Pilates classes are available throughout the country, in venues ranging from specialist studios, with modern versions of Joe Pilates' original equipment, to health clubs, leisure centres, community centres, schools and village halls where the exercises are done mainly on mats. Ask at your local library or leisure centre for a reputable class near you. Searching the internet will tell you all you need to know, and there's a wide range of books and DVDs available for you to practise pilates on your sitting room floor.

For further information on pilates, contact the Pilates Foundation, which claims to be the only not-for-profit professional pilates organisation in the UK dedicated to ensuring the highest standards of training. It does not cover all pilates teachers (telephone 07071 781859; www. pilatesfoundation.com).

Tai chi

This is a mind-body approach to exercise, with many similarities to pilates. But while the latter was invented in New York in the 1920s, tai chi was first performed in China 2,000 years ago and is based on the same Taoist philosophy that gave us acupuncture. Unlike pilates, which is carried out on the floor or special couch, tai chi is done standing up and involves a series of graceful, flowing, balanced, stretching movements. No doubt you've seen people in the park going through the movements and getting strange looks from the swans.

Tai chi increases suppleness and strength, and focuses the mind on position and posture. But, above all, it improves balance. For this reason it has become an important form of exercise to help prevent falls in older people.

Getting started

As with pilates, tai chi classes are held all over the country. Again, it's worth checking that the leader is properly qualified in one of the recognised schools of tai chi. All you need are loose-fitting clothes and bare feet.

There's no official governing body for tai chi. However, there are a number of national commercial organisations set up to establish standards and provide training in one of the several different tai chi disciplines. Check the web or ask at your local leisure centre or library for details of a class near you.

Yoga

This system of mind-body exercises goes back even further than tai chi, originating in India about 5,000 years ago. The most popular form in the West is hatha yoga, which involves sequences of postures or 'asanas' which stretch and flex the body and develop awareness of breathing and relaxation. Meditation is a further refinement for those who wish to use it (see page 107 for advice on using yoga to ease stress).

Yoga is suitable for people of all ages and abilities. Although much of the teaching is in classes, each individual follows their own programme, always remaining within their own limits. It can be very well suited to people with arthritis and other physical ailments or disabilities, and yoga teachers are trained in how to help people with particular problems or difficulties.

Having said that, some yoga classes are very vigorous and quite competitive, so always check with the teacher that the level is appropriate for you, and never feel pressurised into doing something that hurts.

 If your yoga, tai chi or pilates class is of the very relaxed kind, you're probably not getting much in the way of aerobic exercise. In this case you'll need to supplement it with walking, running or other active pursuits to gain all-round fitness and cardiovascular health.

Getting started

Classes, books and DVDs on yoga are available pretty well everywhere. Ask at your local leisure centre or library, or check the web.

 Information on classes can be obtained from the British Wheel of Yoga, which is the governing body for yoga in Great Britain. It has a network of qualified yoga teachers throughout the country (telephone 01529 306851; www.bwy.org.uk).

Small changes, big difference

Being more active begins inside your head. It's about feeling the benefits and joys rather than the barriers. It's about taking every opportunity, no matter how insignificant it may seem, to use your body more. Every little bit of activity helps, so if you're not quite ready to join a class or buy a new set of trainers, why not try some of these easy alternatives:

✓ use the stairs, don't take the lift

✓ get off the bus a stop or two early

✓ stride a little faster up that hill

✓ walk to the shops

✓ do a few minutes stretching on waking every morning

A simple home exercise routine

1 Warm up (about 5 minutes)

Spend about a minute on each of the following. Don't rush them. The key to warming up is slow stretching and toning.

head turns

Stand, feet slightly apart, knees slightly bent (not locked), hands on hips, tummy and bottom tucked in, looking straight ahead, chin up. Without straining, turn your head to the right as far as is comfortable. Hold for a count of three, and return. Then do the same to the left and return. Repeat five times.

elbow circles

Same starting position. Bring your hands up to rest on your shoulders. Bring your elbows up and in to point them straight ahead. Without shrugging your shoulders, raise your elbows as high as is comfortable, and then sweep them slowly round and down again. Repeat five times.

side bends

Stand with your feet shoulder-width apart, arms hanging loose at your sides, facing straight ahead and your tummy and bottom tucked in. Keeping your head and neck in line with your spine, lean *gently* to the left as far as is comfortable. Don't lean forwards or bounce. Hold for a count of three and return to the starting position. Do the same to the right. Repeat five times slowly and gently.

calf stretches

Stand feet together. Keeping your right heel on the floor, place your left foot half a pace in front of you and feel the right calf slightly stretching. Now bend the left knee just enough to feel a little more stretching, as much as is comfortable. Hold for a count of three and return. Do the same with the other leg. Repeat this exercise five times.

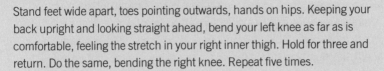
Stand feet wide apart, toes pointing outwards, hands on hips. Keeping your back upright and looking straight ahead, bend your left knee as far as is comfortable, feeling the stretch in your right inner thigh. Hold for three and return. Do the same, bending the right knee. Repeat five times.

2 Stamina-building (minimum 10 minutes)

This is the stamina-building, aerobic, cardiovascular part of the session in which you do a moderately vigorous repetitive exercise that raises your pulse rate and makes you slightly breathless. It could be marching or running on the spot, star jumps, dancing, skipping, step-ups, walking up and down the stairs, going for a brisk walk or run or any combination of these, depending on your inclination and level of fitness.

Whatever you choose, it should be neither uncomfortable nor unpleasant. If you get too puffed or tired, just slow down or rest for a minute or two. Exercising like this, even briefly, is good for you, but for optimum benefit you should try to build up gradually over a few weeks to a steady 20 minutes each session.

You might also like to count your steps by wearing a pedometer, obtainable from sports shops and some pharmacies.

3 Cool down (about 5 minutes)

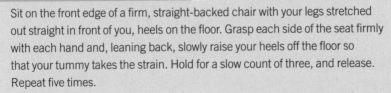
Sit on the front edge of a firm, straight-backed chair with your legs stretched out straight in front of you, heels on the floor. Grasp each side of the seat firmly with each hand and, leaning back, slowly raise your heels off the floor so that your tummy takes the strain. Hold for a slow count of three, and release. Repeat five times.

arm circles

Stand feet slightly apart, knees slightly bent, arms straight out in front of you at shoulder level. Raise your arms slowly above your head, as high and as far back as is comfortable. Hold for three. Then sweep them outwards and backwards, round, down and forwards back to the starting position. Repeat this slowly five times.

side stretches

Stand legs wide apart, toes pointing slightly outwards. Do a thigh stretch to the left and lean head and body to the left, bringing your right arm slowly over your head and stretching as far as is comfortable. Hold for three and return. Do the same to the other side. Repeat five times.

dangles

Stand or move about easily and freely, letting your arms dangle at your sides and shaking yourself loosely like a rag doll. Continue for half a minute – and relax.

That's it. The whole routine shouldn't take you more than 20 or 30 minutes. And if you keep the cardiovascular bit going for 30 minutes it counts as a full day's worth of exercise. Just like that!

Eating well

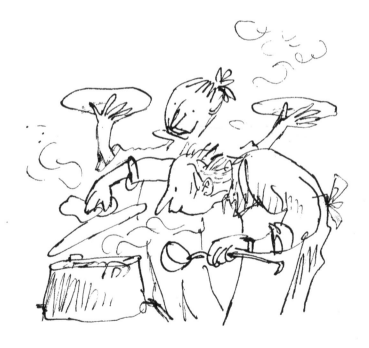

Can there be anything new to say about healthy eating? We're constantly bombarded with messages about the importance of consuming more of this or less of that. Don't we all know that too much fatty, sugary and salty food can kill?

Well, I agree that the basics are pretty well known, but there are still plenty of misconceptions around. This chapter goes through some of these and a few general principles and practicalities. You can always skip the bits you're familiar with.

Let's start with ten common myths.

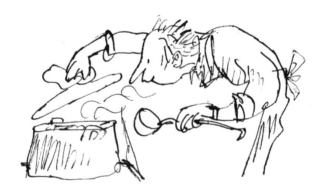

10 myths about healthy eating

Myth 1 Healthy food is boring

What a sad delusion! Just look at the wonderful array of fruit and vegetables in your local supermarket or farmers' market. Feast your eyes on the fresh fish stall. Browse through the delicious low-fat and no-added-sugar products. And look at all those herbs and spices that can add fascinating flavours to your meals. Think Mediterranean, Middle Eastern or Chinese. How can you say that a healthy diet is boring?

Myth 2 Superfoods are superior foods

'Superfoods', a term recently coined in the USA, are foods singled out as being particularly rich sources of vital nutrients such as vitamins, minerals and antioxidants which help to protect against heart disease and cancer. Blueberries, for example, have enjoyed a huge surge of popularity since they've been found to contain high levels of antioxidants. Oats are a good source of fibre and minerals including potassium and magnesium. Spinach is rich in carotenoids (another antioxidant). Walnuts are loaded with omega-3 fatty acids (for a healthy heart). Dark chocolate is packed with flavonoids (yet another antioxidant). And even good old workaday tea (any blend) is infused with these wonderful biochemicals.

But does all this make these foods superior to other foods? The answer is no, not really. OK, they may be full of goodies – but many other foods contain lots of goodies too, particularly fruits, leafy vegetables, grains and pulses. The plain fact is that you can get more of the vital vitamins, minerals and antioxidants than you'll ever need simply by eating a *variety* of healthy foods plucked at random from any supermarket shelf. Why pay silly prices for blueberries flown in from the other side of the world when you can get the same benefit from an apple or two grown in an orchard down the road?

Myth 3 Lean meat is fat-free

Even the leanest meat contains some fat. You may need a magnifying glass to see it, but it's there nestling in among the fibres of flesh. Take a nice deep red lean fillet steak, for instance – about 5 per cent is fat. A skinless chicken breast is saintly by comparison – only about 2 per cent fat. The darker meat in poultry has a little more fat and anything with skin on it is fattier still.

Myth 4 Bread and potatoes are fattening

Not if you avoid smearing the bread with butter or margarine and boil or bake your potatoes rather than fry or roast them. It's the way we cook and eat these starchy carbohydrates that can pile on the calories. Starchy foods provide about the same number of calories, weight for weight, as protein – just over 4 calories per gram. But because, unlike sugar, starch is a 'complex' carbohydrate with very large fluffy molecules, it is much lighter than either sugar or protein and a little goes a long way. In other words, starchy foods like bread, potatoes, rice, pasta, maize and beans are satisfyingly bulky for their weight. You can fill yourself up without overloading yourself with calories so long as you can restrain yourself when it comes to knobs of butter or – horror of horrors – fried bread.

Myth 5 Margarine is less fattening than butter

Unless you choose low-fat margarine, there's no significant difference in calorie content between butter and marge or between 'hard' butter and 'spreadable' butter. They are all about 7 to 8 calories per gram. But low-fat and 'lite' spreads are definitely lower in calories because they are emulsions of fat and water.

Myth 6 Sugar can boost your energy

It depends what you mean by 'energy'. If you mean calorie intake, then, yes, sugar is a sure way to increase your energy intake. Not a great idea if you have a weight problem. Sugar, like starch, is a carbohydrate, providing about 4 calories per gram. However, unlike starch, it is packed into tight little crystals, so it's very easy to have too much of it without realising. If by 'energy' you mean get-up-and-go vitality and verve, then sugary things don't normally have this kind of pick-me-up effect. Indeed, they're more likely to make you feel relaxed and perhaps even sleepy.

Myth 7 Bottled water is healthier than tap water

In terms of purity and safety, most bottled water is no better than the tap water available in developed countries such as Europe or the USA. In fact, many samples of bottled water have been found to have relatively high levels of potentially toxic minerals and bacteria. There are very exacting standards for levels of contaminants and frequency of testing for tap water. The standards for bottled water are much less stringent.

Myth 8 If it's good for you, the more you have of it, the better

Not a great idea. While it's important to eat more healthy things like fruit, vegetables and fish, it's unwise to mainline on any particular food, however healthy it is. The key principles for healthy eating are variety and balance – a range of different types of food and drink and an overall balance between the main food groups.

Myth 9 The experts keep changing their minds

Not so. The basic messages about eating less of the fatty, sugary and salty things, and more fruit and veg, fish and starchy staples, haven't changed for the past 30 years and are consistent across the world.

Of course, there will always be so-called experts who want to push their pet theory about how we've got it all wrong and that they are the first to hit on a whole new way of eating or slimming or living to be 110, and that it's all in their book which has taken America by storm, etc, etc. And of course the media love anything that rocks the establishment, turns accepted wisdom on its head, causes controversy and sells more newspapers. And there will always be a few wacky celebrities whose lives have been transformed by blue-lipped squid sepia sauce or Peruvian purple pomegranate seeds. But don't let these amusing diversions leave you with the impression that the basic healthy eating messages are wrong, because they're not.

Myth 10 A healthy diet is expensive

It doesn't have to be. Remember that processed foods and 'ready meals' tend to be relatively expensive. You can eat a healthy balance of foods without breaking the bank. Semi-skimmed or skimmed milk or low-fat cheeses are about the same price as the full-fat alternatives. It costs less to spread butter more thinly on your toast. Most fruit and vegetables are not expensive, particularly if they're in season. Chicken and turkey are usually cheaper than red meat. Some fish is expensive, but bought once or twice a week it shouldn't make too big a dent in your budget and the canned variety is really quite cheap. Starchy staples – such as rice, potatoes, bread, pulses and cereals – are all modestly priced. If you choose carefully, and avoid too many exotic items flown in from halfway around the world, you can eat very healthily very inexpensively, and help save the planet at the same time.

What is a balanced diet?

We all know we should be eating a 'balanced diet'. But what does this term really mean? Balanced in what way? Rice with peas? Lean with fat? Peaches with cream? Or is it all to do with getting enough protein? Or vitamins and minerals? Or antioxidants?

The whole concept of a balanced diet began back in the days when the biggest problem with our diet was having a shortage of vital nutrients. The most important thing in those days was to make sure that everybody – particularly children, pregnant women, nursing mothers and elderly people – consumed enough energy, protein, vitamins and minerals to keep themselves healthy. And that meant 'balancing' meals by using foods of different types to provide varied sources of essential nutrients.

> **Did you know?** Nutrients are things your body needs to function and can't manufacture itself. They include carbohydrates, proteins and vitamins, and are obtained from food. Nutrients are good for you in the right proportions – fat is actually a nutrient too, and essential to our survival. But, as with all nutrients, it is harmful to have too much.

Today, apart from frail older people living alone, food faddists on crazy diets or people who are ailing for some reason, very few people in the developed world are at risk of undernutrition. We have less real poverty and more reasonably cheap food. Getting enough isn't the problem.

Today's big challenge is overnutrition – eating too much of the wrong things. It's a different kind of imbalance. The diet of the average person today is overloading them in one way or another and putting a strain on certain important body mechanisms.

- **We eat too many calories**. Basically this means putting on weight, which can increase the risk of getting high blood pressure, diabetes and heart disease, not to mention a whole string of other health problems triggered by obesity.

- **We eat too much fat.** Again, this means putting on weight. And high-fat diets also unbalance the fatty substances normally carried in the bloodstream, particularly cholesterol. This can lead to atheroma (fatty deposits on the inner linings of the arteries), which in turn can lead to a heart attack or stroke.

- **We eat too much sugar.** Apart from the calories, this encourages bacteria in the mouth, causing plaque and gum disease and altering the acidity, leading to tooth decay.

- **We eat too much salt.** This can push up the blood pressure and increase the risk of heart disease, stroke and chronic kidney disease.

There are some things, however, that the average person today does not get enough of:

- **Too** little **dietary fibre.** Roughage, as it is also known, is mainly found in wholegrain cereals, wholemeal bread, fruit and vegetables. It eases the passage of food residue through the intestines, helps prevent constipation, and reduces the risk of disorders such as piles, diverticulosis and bowel cancer. It also aids the digestion and absorption of sugars and fats, thus helping to control blood sugar and cholesterol levels.

- **Too** few **antioxidants.** These are found in fruit, salads, green leafy vegetables and eggs. Antioxidants are vitamins and minerals that help our body deal with the damaging effects of so-called 'free radicals' – the by-products of cell activity that hasten ageing, heart disease and cancer. Vitamins A, C and E are antioxidants. So are selenium and zinc.

While we're on the subject of the balanced diet, there's another general principle I should mention. You need to think in terms of your whole diet – everything you eat and drink over a period of time, say a week. People can get so finicky about individual food items that they lose sight of what their diet as a whole is doing for their health. They can't see the wood for the trees. They think that this or that item is either 'good' or 'bad', 'fattening' or 'slimming', and either eat as much of it as they can or avoid it like the plague.

It may be easy to categorise food and drink in this black and white way, but it misses the important point about the totality of the diet being what really counts. To tuck into a buttered bun or plate of bacon and eggs is not another nail in your coffin, as long as you generally cut down on fatty things to compensate.

Did you know? A calorie is a measurement of energy, or 'heat'. The calories in the food you eat give you the energy you need to live. If you take in more calories than you use up, you will gain weight. One pound of fat contains about 3,500 calories, so if you eat 3,500 more calories than your body needs, you will gain a pound.

The balance of good health

So far I've been talking about nutrients, but what about actual food? When you're trundling your trolley round the aisles, you're probably not thinking fat, sugar, salt, fibre, vitamins and minerals. You may check the odd label for calorie content, saturated fat or sodium, but you're much more likely to be thinking potatoes, cereals, sausages, cheese, eggs, milk, onions, carrots, apples, chicken, bananas, yoghurt, baked beans, fish fingers or any one of a zillion other items of food and drink.

The Plate of Good Health

About one-third of your diet should comprise fruit and vegetables, one-third starchy staples, and one-third should be a combination of protein and dairy foods. Fatty snacks and sugary things should make up a very small proportion. Here's a useful way to picture it. The size of each segment indicates the proportion from each category you should aim for over a period of time, say a week.

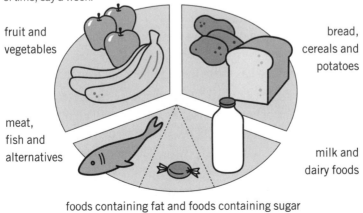

fruit and vegetables

bread, cereals and potatoes

meat, fish and alternatives

milk and dairy foods

foods containing fat and foods containing sugar

What's so unhealthy about unhealthy eating?

There's a long list of diseases and disorders that can be brought on by years of eating the wrong balance of food and drink. Let's look at just a few of the depressing diagnoses that might await someone who has eaten a typical British diet for far too long – fried foods, tinned vegetables, salty snacks, cakes and biscuits, all washed down with buckets of sugary tea and carbonated drinks.

Obesity

A high-fat, high-sugar diet is loaded with calories and is bound to lead to overweight or obesity. About one middle-aged person in three is obese. Apart from increasing the risk of high blood pressure, diabetes, heart disease and stroke, obesity aggravates back trouble, arthritis, foot problems and gallstones. It can also hinder recovery from surgery, with a higher risk of complications. Last but not least, obesity can make people very unhappy.

High blood pressure

High blood pressure is also known as hypertension, but not because of its link with stress. We all need some blood pressure – it's what pushes our blood around our bodies. With each beat of our heart, another wave of pressure can be felt as a pulse in our arteries. Like all waves, it has a peak and a trough. The peak pressure is called 'systolic' and the trough pressure is called 'diastolic'. Blood pressure is measured as these two numbers, for example, 120/80.

Problems begin when our blood pressure is raised too high. This increases our risk of heart disease, stroke, chronic kidney disease and damage to the retinas of our eyes. High blood pressure is a very common problem among older people. It is often known as the 'silent killer' because it causes virtually no symptoms itself – its effects are only seen when something awful happens as a consequence.

Why do so many people have high blood pressure? There are several reasons, but the most common causes are:

- too much salt in the diet
- being overweight
- over-indulgence in alcohol
- lack of exercise
- chronic stress
- a genetic tendency (it tends to run in families and is more common among black people)

Cutting down on salt, drinking moderately, staying slim and exercising regularly can all help to keep your resting blood pressure down and preclude the need for medication.

> **Did you know?** Blood pressure tends to rise as we get older. Until recently, this was thought to be part of normal ageing. But studies in a number of developing countries have shown that the average healthy person's blood pressure remains fairly low throughout life, at around 110/70. This suggests that our rising blood pressure is largely due to our relatively high salt intake. It should not go above 140/90 at any age.

Coronary heart disease

Heart attacks and angina are usually caused by the coronary arteries in the heart becoming clogged with fatty deposits. These deposits consist mainly of cholesterol and are more likely to occur if there's a high level of cholesterol in the bloodstream.

Most of this cholesterol is made in the liver, using the building blocks of fat absorbed from our food, and is transported by the bloodstream to tissues all over the body where it plays a vital part in the workings of our cell membranes. Unfortunately, over the years, it can silt up the arteries, especially where these are narrow and tortuous, as in the heart and brain. The higher the level of this cholesterol in the blood, the greater the risk of clogged arteries, angina, heart attacks and strokes, although other risk factors such as high blood pressure and smoking are important too.

This clog-prone cholesterol is a type called low-density lipoprotein or LDL cholesterol, popularly known as 'bad' cholesterol for obvious reasons. This is the cholesterol that's too high in most of us, mostly because we're eating too much saturated fat in our food.

There's another type of cholesterol in the blood called high-density lipoprotein (or HDL cholesterol). This cholesterol is on its way back to the liver to be dismantled. Interestingly, a high level of HDL cholesterol in the blood is associated with a reduction in the risk of angina, heart attacks and strokes. It is therefore known as 'good' cholesterol.

 Choose skimmed or semi-skimmed milk. Cut the visible fat off meat and choose leaner portions. If you're a vegetarian, have plenty of nuts and seeds. Replace palm oil or blended vegetable oil with an oil high in unsaturated fats, such as sunflower or olive oil.

Needless to say, the balance between these two types of cholesterol in the bloodstream is crucial to a person's long-term health and we should all be doing our best to keep our LDL cholesterol down and our HDL cholesterol up. The way to achieve this is by cutting down on saturated fats (and trans fats), partially replacing them with unsaturated fats, and by taking regular aerobic exercise. How well we're succeeding can be revealed by a simple blood test (blood lipid profile) or the rather more perilous approach of waiting to see whether we get angina or have a heart attack or stroke.

Stroke

This is a 'brain attack', caused either by a clot lodging in one of the arteries to the brain (thrombotic stroke) or by internal bleeding from an artery within or surrounding the brain (haemorrhagic stroke).

Types of fat

✗ saturated fats

These mainly come from animal sources (for example, milk, cream, butter, cheese, red meat and meat products). They also include some plant oils (for example, palm oil and coconut oil). Saturated fats raise the level of 'bad' cholesterol in the bloodstream and increase the risk of heart disease and stroke. We should try to cut down on them.

✓ unsaturated fats

These are divided into monounsaturated fats, which are mainly found in plants and poultry (for example, avocados, olive oil, rapeseed oil, chicken fat), and polyunsaturated fats, which are mainly found in plants and fish (for example, sunflower oil, oily fish). Unsaturated fats help to raise the level of 'good' cholesterol in the bloodstream. We should try to eat more of them.

✗ trans fats

These are usually created artificially by partial hydrogenation of unsaturated fats (for example, hydrogenated vegetable oil). Hydrogenation is a process whereby liquid vegetable oil is converted into solid or semi-solid fat (shortening), which is commonly used in baking. Trans fats are found in hard margarines, deep-fried foods, pastries, cakes and biscuits. Trans fats are even more likely to produce 'bad' cholesterol than saturated fats. We should try to cut out trans fats altogether.

Both types are more likely to occur in older people, especially if they have high blood pressure, high cholesterol or they smoke.

You can minimise the risk of stroke by eating a balanced diet and cutting down on foods that contain 'bad' cholesterol and salt.

Moderate exercise, moderate drinking and absolutely no smoking all play their part too.

Diabetes

Contrary to popular belief, eating too much sugar doesn't cause diabetes – not directly anyway. However, type 2 diabetes, the usual form in older people, is more likely to occur if you're overweight, so going easy on the calories and keeping active can help to keep it at bay.

People who already have diabetes should make sure they are aware of the sugary things in their diet: sugar can make their blood glucose level rise too high very quickly, which can lead to complications, including, in some cases, diabetic coma.

In general, people with diabetes should follow the same principles of healthy eating as anyone else. But it's particularly important that they have three regular meals a day – no skipping breakfast or lunch – and that these are well spaced out to help to keep their blood glucose under control.

Each meal should include starchy foods, which have a low glycaemic index (low GI). Unlike sugar, these are slowly absorbed into the system. Good choices include grainy breads such as granary, pumpernickel or rye, pasta (especially wholewheat), basmati, brown or easy-cook rice, new potatoes, sweet potato, yam, porridge oats and bran cereals.

There's absolutely no need to buy special 'diabetic' foods or drinks. They offer no particular benefit and are not cheap.

Bowel disorders

As we sail through middle age our bowels can often be a cause of discomfort or embarrassment. We get constipation, wind, irritable bowel, or the nasty gripes of diverticular disease. And there's always the risk of bowel cancer, which is much more common in older people.

Our diet has a profound effect on our bowels, both in the short term and over a period of years. Many of our problems are caused by a lack of fibre in our food – what used to be called roughage, but might be better thought of as 'smoothage' because it smoothes the progress of food residue through the bowels by absorbing water and giving the motions enough softness and bulk for the colon to get a grip and speed things along. So high-fibre foods – oats, high-bran cereals, pulses, fruit and leafy or root vegetables – are important for a healthy bowel. There's also evidence that a diet lower in fat and red meat may help to reduce the risk of cancer of the colon and rectum.

Irritable bowel is more complicated and may be triggered by a high-fibre diet. Here the problem is thought to be a disturbance of the normal healthy bacteria that live in the large bowel. The condition may be helped by eating live yoghurt to restore the natural balance.

Healthy eating – the basics

Getting confused by all this dietary advice? Well, there's no need to be because the good news is that the same healthy diet reduces the risk of developing all of these conditions. By an amazing quirk of good fortune, or perhaps the benign influence of Mother Nature, the balance of foods we need to help us stay slim, for example, is exactly the same as that which helps us avoid diabetes and prevents heart disease, strokes and bowel cancer. Imagine the confusion if we had to choose between different diets according to the particular disease we were trying to avoid. We don't. We just need to stick to the basics.

So let's get down to the nitty gritty. How do these broad healthy eating principles translate into what food and drink we should choose? Well, this is the easy part. These are my six golden rules, based on guidelines from no less an authority than the World Health Organization (WHO). They're sensible, simple and practical, and shouldn't add more to your shopping bill.

1 Eat more fruit, vegetables and salads

Fruit and vegetables contain lots of healthy fibre and vital vitamins and minerals, especially when eaten raw or lightly cooked. The WHO recommends a *minimum* of 400g (just under 1lb) of fruit and vegetables a day, not counting potatoes, which are in the starchy food category. That's at least five average sized pieces or portions of fruit or vegetables every day. Fruit juice can count as one of the five. Tinned and frozen fruit and vegetables and dried fruit also count. But it's best to eat fresh fruit or raw or lightly cooked vegetables, well washed, as cooking can destroy some of their nutrients. About one-third of what we eat should be fruit and vegetables.

2 Eat more starchy foods, such as bread, potatoes, pasta, rice, cereals, beans and lentils

These are the starchy staples that should be a major part of our daily diet. Like fruit and vegetables, they should make up about a third of what we eat, providing 50 to 70 per cent of our calorie intake – about double the amount the average person eats at present. Wholemeal or wholegrain versions of these foods are best because they retain all the vitamins, minerals and fibre which would otherwise be lost in the process of refining.

3 Limit meat and dairy products, eggs and cooking oil

The main concerns are the calories and saturated fats in these foods. The WHO recommends that we should derive no more than about one-third of our total calories from fats and oils of any kind. And, of those, only about a third should be from saturated fats. That means cutting down on fatty meats, meat products and full-fat dairy products.

The WHO also recommends cutting trans fats to as near zero as possible. This means avoiding anything cooked in hydrogenated vegetable oil and hydrogenated fat, including lard and hard margarine. We do of course need some fats and oils in our diet (not least because they often contain fat-soluble vitamins – A, D, E and K). But we should make sure that most of these fats are mono- or polyunsaturated. In other words we should choose things cooked with corn oil, sunflower oil, olive oil or safflower oil and eat poultry and oily fish more often.

4 Cut down on sugary things

Sugar is a concentrated form of calories – 4 per seductively crystalline gram – but has no other nutritional value. Eating or drinking sugary things frequently can encourage oral plaque (mouth bacteria), leading to bad breath, gum disease, tooth decay and weight gain. We have no need whatsoever for the refined sugar contained in sweets, cakes, biscuits, ice cream and sugary drinks, and it should provide no more than about 10 per cent of our calorie intake.

5 Cut down on salty things

Salt is no longer the precious commodity it used to be (Roman soldiers were paid in salt, hence the word 'salary'). Today it's as cheap as it is tasty and, on average, we eat about ten times more of it than our body actually needs. Salt is everywhere – in bread, cereals, processed foods, savoury snacks, canned vegetables, not to mention the salt we use in cooking and shake over our chips. The trouble is that all this salt can really push up our blood pressure, which becomes a significant problem as we get older. We need to cut down from the current average of about 9 grams a day to no more than 6 grams a day. The easiest way to do this is to gradually wean ourselves off it – add less and less to food, replace it with lemon juice and other seasonings, and avoid obviously salty things like anchovies and salted peanuts.

6 Eat chicken, turkey and fish

Chicken, turkey, guinea fowl, duck and goose are much less fatty than red meat. Most of the fat in poultry is monounsaturated and is found in the skin and liver. However, the dark meat is a little fattier than the white.

As far as fish is concerned, most of us should eat more of it. Apart from being an excellent source of protein, fish also contains essential vitamins and minerals. White fish, such as cod, haddock, plaice and whiting, is very low in fat. Oily fish, such as sardines, pilchards, mackerel, herring and salmon, is by definition quite fatty, but the fat is mostly a polyunsaturated form known as 'omega-3', which is good for the heart and arteries as well as the brain and nervous system. Oily fish are also good sources of vitamins A and D.

The livers of some white fish contain high levels of oil (for example, cod liver oil, halibut liver oil), which contain vitamins A, D and omega-3s. These are powerful nutrients with lots of health benefits – they may even reduce the risk of coronary heart disease. Go for a reputable brand of fish oil (less likely to contain pollutants) and don't exceed the stated dose.

The recommendation for most people is to eat one or two portions of fish a week, preferably alternating white fish with oily fish.

> **Did you know?** It might surprise you to know that we eat on average ten times more salt than we need. And another fact: the body doesn't need any refined sugar at all.

Fish for health

Fish is good for our health. We should eat one or two portions a week, preferably alternating white fish with oily fish.

oily fish	white fish	
tuna (fresh)	tuna (tinned)	flounder
salmon	cod	hake
trout	haddock	john dory
mackerel	plaice	monkfish
herring	coley	red / grey
sardines	whiting	mullet
pilchards	lemon sole	snapper
kippers	skate	sea bass
eel	halibut	sea bream
whitebait	rock salmon	marlin
anchovies	catfish	
swordfish	shark	
bloaters	turbot	
sprats	dover sole	

Fresh tuna is oily and full of omega-3s, but when it's canned it loses most of its oil (even if olive oil is added to the can) and becomes more like white fish.

Vitamins, minerals and antioxidants

These words are often bandied about when people talk about diet and nutrition. But if you're eating a balanced diet with plenty of fruit and vegetables, you're almost certainly getting all the goodies you need. For more information, read on.

Vitamins – how important are they?

In a word, they're vital – hence the name. Vitamins don't provide any calories or raw materials, but they act as catalysts or biochemical lubricants, enabling various processes to take place. Each vitamin has its own particular part to play in our body chemistry. Although a particular vitamin may only be needed in tiny quantities, a lack of it could eventually lead to one of the 'deficiency' diseases, such as scurvy (lack of vitamin C) or pellagra (lack of niacin or vitamin B3).

There are two main families of vitamin: fat-soluble and water-soluble. Fat-soluble vitamins (A, D, E and K) are mainly found in fatty foods, mostly from animal sources, and are stored in the liver for use when necessary, so a daily intake isn't required. However, these stores can build up to quite high levels, so they may be harmful if taken in excess.

By contrast, water-soluble vitamins (all the others, including the B vitamins and vitamin C, mostly found in plant sources such as cereals, green leafy vegetables and fruit) can't be stored at all and any excess consumed is quickly removed in the urine. So, while overdosing on water-soluble vitamins is impossible, this also means that you need to take in fresh supplies every day. And 'fresh' means fresh because, unlike fat-soluble vitamins, water-soluble vitamins are destroyed by cooking and by being exposed to air.

To retain as many vitamins as possible, fruit and vegetables should be eaten fresh and raw, or cooked quickly and lightly (for example, steamed or stir-fried).

What about minerals and trace elements?

In a similar way to vitamins, there are several minerals and trace elements essential to the normal working of our body chemistry. They are needed to control the movement of body fluids inside and outside cells, turn the food we eat into energy, and build strong bones and teeth. Examples of essential minerals include sodium, potassium, calcium, magnesium, iron, phosphorus, and sulphur. The main ones we need to boost are calcium, magnesium and iron.

Trace elements are essential minerals needed in very tiny quantities. Here are the main ones (in alphabetical order): boron, chromium, cobalt, copper, fluoride, iodine, manganese, molybdenum, selenium, silicon and zinc.

A balanced diet should provide all the essential minerals and trace elements most of us need. But supplements might help people with particular conditions such as iron-deficiency, anaemia or osteoporosis (where calcium is essential).

What are antioxidants?

We hear quite a lot about these wonder nutrients with apparently magical powers to prevent cancer and heart disease. But what are they? Can they really save your life?

Well, the science behind this is pretty complex, but the short answer is that they are mainly plant-derived nutrients that have the potential to reduce the damage done by so-called 'free radicals' in the body. These free radicals are every bit as troublesome and disruptive as they sound. They are highly reactive biochemical by-products of normal cell activity with a powerful oxidising effect that can interfere with dozens of bodily processes. For example, there's increasing evidence that, in the walls of our arteries, free radicals hasten the formation of cholesterol-laden deposits (atheroma) leading to clogging and thrombosis. And they cause other changes that predispose to certain cancers, such as bowel cancer.

Eating antioxidant-rich foods helps to prevent, slow down or even reverse the damaging and dangerous effects of free radicals. They may even help to decelerate the process of ageing.

So how do we recognise an antioxidant when we see one? Well, they include some very familiar nutrients: vitamins A, C and E, for instance – the famous 'ACE' trio so beloved of the nutritional supplement industry; and beta-carotene, a plant-derived precursor of vitamin A. Some minerals too, such as selenium and manganese, are antioxidants. These are also widely found in plants.

One of the main reasons for eating more fruit and vegetables, as well as wholegrains, nuts and pulses, is to make sure we get dozens of antioxidants. More join the list every day: lycopene in ripe tomatoes, tannin in red wine and tea, eugenol in clove, basil and cinnamon, bioflavonoids in blackcurrants and pomegranates, myricetin in walnuts, and so on and so on.

But there's no need to pore over the labels in the health food store looking for the ultimate antioxidant. The basic message is very simple: eat plenty of fruit and vegetables (well washed and preferably organic), plus wholegrains, nuts and pulses, and you'll get all the antioxidants you need.

Who needs extra vitamins and minerals?

It's pretty clear from everything we've said so far that, providing we eat a good, well-balanced and varied diet, and follow the basic healthy eating principles on pages 63–66, we shouldn't need to take any nutritional supplements. Most of us can rely completely on what is, after all, the most natural approach to good nutritional health – food.

Nevertheless, some people may benefit from a boost of extra vitamins and minerals. If you're recovering from a recent illness or operation, for example. Or if you're feeling run down for any reason. Or you've lost your appetite or your energy. Or perhaps if you have difficulty getting to the shops to buy a healthy variety of foods. Or you're feeling so depressed you just can't get it together enough to make yourself a nutritious meal. Over-the-counter multivitamins and minerals aren't cheap, but they may help to supplement an otherwise inadequate diet in people who are debilitated for these sorts of reasons. Choose a multivitamin and mineral formulation containing vitamins C and B complex and iron.

But far too many people pay huge amounts of money for nutritional supplements they don't need. Some believe that extra vitamins and minerals on top of a healthy diet will bring some kind of super-health, although there's no evidence for this. Indeed, there are dangers in overdosing on many of these micronutrients. Others use the taking of supplements as an excuse to stop bothering about healthy eating – always a mistake. And others still become so convinced that they're in dire need of some particular micronutrient, even though it may be present in a wide range of foods, that they 'mainline' on it – popping pills to get their fix of biotin or boron or some obscure co-enzyme that's all too often destroyed by their digestive juices before it gets beyond the stomach.

Functional foods

A major commercial trend in the last few years has been the marketing of foods that purport to have a therapeutic effect in helping to prevent or ameliorate some medical condition. Examples of these so-called 'functional foods' include breads with vitamin and mineral supplements or added fibre, margarines which contain a balance of fats to boost HDL cholesterol ('good' cholesterol), and yoghurts containing 'probiotics' (dairy bacteria thought to stabilise the natural bacteria in the intestines in people with irritable bowel syndrome).

Many of these foods can have a potentially beneficial effect for people with particular health problems, although, again, the same benefits can usually be achieved through a healthy, balanced and varied diet.

Why choose organic?

Organic food is booming. More and more of us are choosing to pay that little bit more for produce that is grown free of pesticides or artificial fertilisers and stored without artificial preservatives. Or for organic milk, eggs, meat and fish from stock reared without antibiotics or hormones.

As far as your health is concerned, the main advantage of choosing organic is that you can be reasonably sure that you're avoiding traces of these artificial substances, particularly if you happen to be allergic or sensitive to them.

There are some drawbacks – the main ones being that your fruit and veg are more likely to be blemished and have a shorter shelf-life. But I reckon organic foods taste so much nicer that it's worth putting up with a little inconvenience. And anyway they're much kinder to wildlife and the countryside.

Making sense of the labels

The food industry is catching on to the fact that consumers want to know more about the good and bad effects of the food they eat. There's also pressure from government and lobby groups to make this information available. Look out for the two main food-labelling styles described here.

1 **The traffic-light scheme** is very simple. Products are given red, amber or green 'lights', according to whether the proportions of fat, saturated fat, sugar and salt are rated high, medium or low by nationally agreed criteria. This system was developed by the Food Standards Agency and has been adopted by a number of supermarket chains. It is helpful when choosing between broad food categories, although not quite so helpful when trying to discriminate between, say, different types of pizza or pork pie.

2 But some parts of the food industry prefer **the rival GDA (guidance daily amount) system** which simply gives a set of percentages representing the contribution a portion of the food makes to an average adult's daily allowance of fat, saturated fat, sugar, salt, and calories.

This sounds very useful on the face of it, but there are snags. One is that quite a lot of people don't really understand percentages. Another is that the GDAs are for an 'average adult' and very few of us fit that category – we're usually men (higher GDAs), women (lower GDAs) or children (much lower GDAs). And there are further complications such as being pregnant, breastfeeding or trying to lose weight. So, even if you can work out the percentages, the figures don't really apply. All of which is very confusing.

 For more information visit the Food Standards Agency website (www.food.gov.uk).

Small changes, big difference

It may be a cliché to say 'you are what you eat', but it also happens to be true. Although our body is remarkably adept at extracting the goodness from our daily diet, it can all too easily take on board far too much of the wrong stuff.

That's why I can't emphasise enough the importance of a balanced diet. I hope by now you realise how simple and straightforward healthy eating can be, and that it doesn't mean you can't enjoy your food, or treat yourself on occasion.

However for some people it can be very difficult to change old, bad habits.

If this is you, then remember that change can come about gradually. So why not pick something from the list on the following page and do it this week: that way you'll be making a small improvement to your diet straightaway.

Feeling good!

- ✓ cut down on cheese
- ✓ substitute brown bread for white
- ✓ fry with olive, sunflower or corn oil
- ✓ skim surface fat off casseroles and pot-roasts
- ✓ cook with a microwave to preserve flavour and nutrients
- ✓ use less salt and more lemon juice, herbs and spices
- ✓ use fresh or dried fruit to sweeten desserts
- ✓ steam leafy vegetables
- ✓ use fresh fruit and raw or lightly cooked vegetables
- ✓ grill or bake meat and fish
- ✓ cook something wicked once a week!

Watching your weight

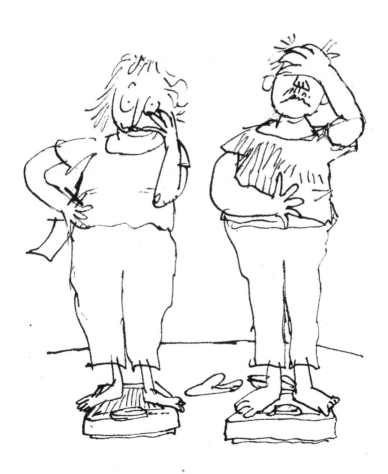

Yes, it's a constant struggle. Yes, it's dispiriting. Yes, it seems to get harder not easier. You do all the right things – say no to biscuits, fend off chocolates, spurn puddings, deny yourself all sorts of treats – and yet you still put on weight. You spend mealtime after mealtime nibbling zero-calorie crispbreads and chasing a few lettuce leaves around a plate, and yet you just can't shift those love handles. Is there any hope?

Well, yes there is. Middle age doesn't have to mean middle-aged spread, and more spare time doesn't have to mean more spare tyre. I'm not promising a new fat-busting wonder drug, nor yet another miracle diet. I'm simply saying that there are ways that can help you to tip the scales towards weight loss rather than weight gain, some of which you may not have tried. If you can arrange your life so that you lose just one pound a week, or even half of that, you'll be winning, albeit rather slowly. The secret is not to expect too much too soon. Lasting weight loss takes time and patience.

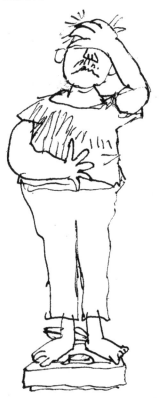

Weight gain in middle age

Why do people put on weight as they get older?

Well, as we all know, we put on weight when we consume more calories than we burn up. So, if we find ourselves with an ever-expanding waistline or needing a larger dress size, it can only be because we're being less careful about how many calories we eat and drink or, more likely, we're not burning them up as efficiently as we did in our younger days. Perhaps we're a bit less active than we were or our metabolism has slowed down slightly. Or perhaps we've reached a stage in life when we can indulge in longer, heavier meals or have more frequent snacks.

For whatever reason, it doesn't take much to tip the balance towards obesity. Indeed, it has been estimated that the average adult whose daily energy input is just 60 calories more than their energy output will become obese over a period of 10 years. That's the equivalent of just half a slice of bread a day more than your body needs. It's not surprising that chubbiness has a habit of creeping up on us.

Glow-worm or cold fish?

There's another reason why it often becomes harder to keep our weight under control as we get older – our bodies become less efficient at turning excess calories into heat. This is known as thermogenesis. Every time we eat a meal, some of the calories are used to make us just a little warmer for an hour or two afterwards instead of being stored as body fat. However, the number of calories used to generate heat after eating varies greatly from person to person.

The lucky ones among us are 'glow-worms' – they produce quite a lot of heat, which they dissipate through their skin, and they manage to stay slim with little apparent effort. The less fortunate are the 'cold fish', who have poor thermogenesis. They only have to look at a cream cake to pile on the pounds. Most people are somewhere in between. In general, men tend towards the glow-worm end of the spectrum and women towards the cold fish end. Younger people tend to be glow-worms, older people cold fish. However, there's some good news if you happen to be a bit of a cold fish: regular exercise can help to shift your metabolism up a gear towards the glow-worm category. Perhaps not much, but it might be just enough to tip the balance.

 You don't have to work all that hard to burn calories. Twenty minutes of brisk walking should offset that shortbread finger at tea-time.

What's so unhealthy about being overweight?

But what is so awful about being a bit chubby? Surely it's better to be plump than miserable.

If it were merely a matter of chubbiness I'd agree. But being overweight, whether by a lot or just a little, has significant implications for health, especially for the over-fifties. But don't feel downhearted. We'll skip quickly through the scary stuff and then look at some of the ways that you can start to turn things around.

Heart disease, stroke and diabetes

The bad news is that even a few excess pounds can increase your likelihood of developing high blood pressure and push up the level of fats, including LDL cholesterol ('bad' cholesterol), in your blood. These effects together add significantly to your risk of heart disease or a stroke (see page 59).

Being overweight also makes it more likely you'll develop a resistance to insulin which can lead to type 2 diabetes, another powerful risk factor for these cardiovascular catastrophes.

And once your chubbiness takes you into the obesity bracket, your risk of getting angina, suffering a heart attack or stroke, or developing type 2 diabetes is doubled or trebled.

Metabolic syndrome

The most worrying form of obesity in this respect is so-called 'central' obesity – an increased waist circumference, or a fat tummy to you and me. This 'apple' shape (in contrast to the 'pear' shape of big hips and thighs) is linked to a whole bunch of cardiovascular risk factors. These include high blood pressure, high blood glucose, high blood triglyceride (a fatty substance) and low HDL cholesterol ('good' cholesterol) associated with resistance to the hormone insulin.

This package of ill effects is collectively known as the metabolic syndrome, and the metabolic syndrome is worrying because it carries a much higher risk of progressing to heart disease, stroke and type 2 diabetes. Needless to say, men are more likely than women to become big 'apples', which partly explains their greater vulnerability to heart disease in middle age. So are people from certain ethnic backgrounds, notably south Asians.

Internal fat

Recent studies using MRI (magnetic resonance imaging) scanning have shown that many older people have far too much fatty tissue around vital internal organs such as the heart and liver. This internal fat is strongly linked to the metabolic syndrome I've just talked about. The startling thing is that it can even be present in people who look slim. It's difficult to measure without sophisticated equipment, but most people over 50 can assume they are harbouring too much of the stuff in their internal nooks and crannies, particularly within their abdomen.

Unfortunately, this type of fat seems to be rather diet-proof and difficult to shift simply by restricting calorie intake or fat consumption. But the good news is that it does seem to respond to exercise – an active lifestyle can help to melt it away. Yet another reason to keep moving, especially in our later years.

And the list goes on ...

There's a long list of other ills that might be triggered or aggravated by obesity. These include:

- gallbladder disease
- sleep apnoea (interference with breathing rhythm at night)
- arthritic pain
- back trouble
- cancer of the colon
- depression
- risk of complications after surgery

So the potential misery of not doing something about your cheery chubbiness far outweighs the relatively minor inconvenience of making a truly determined and sustained effort to tackle it.

But we shouldn't just focus on these big health issues. Most people suffer a general sense of discomfort from being overweight. We can't walk as fast or as far as we like; we can't get out of a chair so easily; we don't enjoy shopping for new clothes and we never run for that bus. If we're playing with kids or grandchildren we go red in the face, and if we're going for a walk we have to stop and look at the view rather too often. Conversely, those times when we have lost weight – whether through a disciplined diet and exercise regime or two weeks on holiday in a country where the food didn't quite agree with us – haven't we all felt noticeably lighter, faster and, in fact, *happier?*

So there really are a great number of reasons why we should lose some of that extra weight. And the chances are that you can really make progress, even if you've tried and failed many times before. Perhaps you were expecting too much too soon, or simply weren't using the right combination of changes for long enough to see results. There are plenty of small lifestyle changes you can make that will really help. Becoming a little bit more active and eating a little more healthily will – slowly but surely – lead to a huge improvement in the way you look and feel.

What is obesity?

Clearly, 'obesity' is more than just being a bit overweight. Until now, I've used both terms. Now is the time to work out which applies to you. In fact, the terms 'overweight' and 'obese' have strict definitions. You might be surprised how easily you can slip into the obese bracket – perhaps a lot more easily than you can slip into your favourite jeans.

It's easy to work out whether you're in the overweight or obese bracket, so I don't want you closing the book because it's all getting too complicated. All you need know are your weight, height and waist size. This will allow you to assess your body fatness (sometimes called adiposity) in just a few minutes. See page 83.

You and your weight

Your weight depends to some extent on your height – the taller you are, the more you can weigh without being overweight, and vice versa. Both measurements are needed to calculate a formula for your fatness. The most widely used formula is the Body Mass Index, or BMI. Technically, this is your weight in kilos divided by the square of your height in metres (kg/m^2).

 You can calculate your BMI quickly and easily at www.bbc.co.uk/health. Click on 'healthy living' and go to the 'your weight' section.

Your BMI correlates quite well with the amount of body fat you're carrying around, not only in the obvious places, but also hidden in the cavities and recesses of your interior. According to the World Health Organization (WHO), adults with a BMI of 18.5 to 24.9 are a healthy weight; those with a score of between 25 and 29.9 are overweight; and those with BMI of 30 to 39.9 are obese. A person with a BMI of 40 or more is 'severely obese'. These categories correspond to the bands in the height-weight chart on page 83.

However your BMI doesn't tell the whole story. For one thing it doesn't allow for the fact that some people, men mainly, may be quite muscular and can be quite heavy without being fat. Nor is it useful in assessing where any excess fat is – in other words, whether you're an 'apple' or a 'pear', which as we saw on page 79 can be important in determining your risk of the problems associated wth the metabolic syndrome.

For those reasons, your doctor or nurse may measure your waist size as well as your BMI. And of course you can easily check it for yourself by measuring your waist at the level of your tummy button. Don't hold in. Just stand there and relax.

Your risk of problems increases gradually with a widening girth. If you're a woman, it's significantly higher at 32 inches (80cm) and much higher at 35 inches (88cm). For men, the equivalent measurements are 37 inches (94cm) and 40 inches (102cm).

Target weight

The weight you should aim for will depend on how overweight you are. If you're moderately overweight, you should aim to get down eventually to the healthy range for your height (see page 83). But if you're more than mildly obese, then it's better to aim for a more modest reduction – say, 10 per cent of your current weight. This will bring considerable health benefits, although you may still be over your designated healthy range. But every little helps. Even a 5 per cent reduction, if you can keep your weight down, is beneficial.

When to weigh yourself

It's all too easy to become obsessed by your weight, perhaps checking it every day or, if you're really in deep, two or three times a day. This is completely unnecessary and could rapidly turn you into a slimming bore. It may also make you feel discouraged about your situation and more likely to give up. Everybody's weight pops up and down from day to day and throughout each day, depending mainly on how much fluid is taken into the stomach, how much is retained in tissues and how much has been eliminated from the system. These fluid fluctuations may show up fleetingly on

Check your weight here

Weigh yourself once a week without clothes. Check your weight against your height (without shoes) by running your finger up the column for your weight until it reaches the horizontal row for your height, and check the diagonal band that you're in.

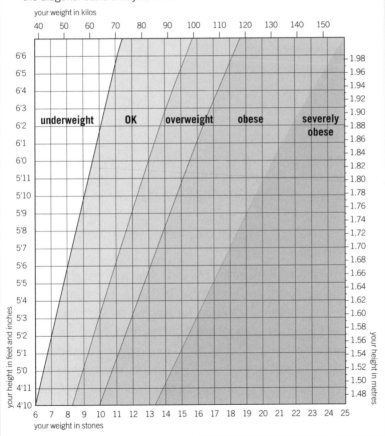

your bathroom scales but mean nothing so far as your body fat is concerned.

Shifting fat is a much more gradual process. It can take up to a week for the calories in that cream cake you've just scoffed to be converted into extra inches on your hips or waist, and just as long for any reduction in calories to release excess body fat. I'm oversimplifying of course because, in reality, laying down and releasing body fat is a continuous two-way process. The net change is very gradual and there's absolutely no point in weighing yourself more than once a week, preferably at the same time of day. What you're measuring is the result of a week's worth of eating, drinking and exercising. If you do have a slightly obsessive nature, you can usefully channel it into keeping a chart of your weekly progress (see page 88).

How to get slimmer and stay slimmer

You hear so many conflicting stories. Some people swear by the Atkins diet or the Pritikin diet. Others mainline on grapefruit or pomegranates or whichever is the latest allegedly fat-banishing wonder ingredient. Still others say it's all about eating foods in the right combination. And then there's the view that diets don't work at all, or even make you fatter.

The truth is really quite simple and rather mundane. To lose weight successfully – and to maintain that weight loss and stay slimmer – requires a makeover in the way you eat and drink and move your body. It's not about going on this or that diet: it's about making a number of small changes to your ordinary everyday eating and drinking habits. And it's not about throwing yourself into a punishing exercise programme: it's about gently and gradually becoming a little more active in your everyday life. These are small changes that can make a big difference. You won't see instant and

Pears and cellulite

A huge and very lucrative myth has grown up around the idea of cellulite. The term was invented to describe the dimpled fatty tissue that women tend to have on their hips and thighs. The theory is that it's a kind of rogue fat caused by unknown 'toxins' and that it's somehow unnatural. More important, many women consider it unsightly and somehow to be eliminated.

The awkward truth is that there's nothing special about this so-called cellulite. It's the natural fatty tissue that women are heir to. Female hormones give women a pear-shaped distribution of fat, which, as we've seen, is less likely than the male apple shape to cause health problems in middle age. In evolutionary terms, it probably represents a last-ditch store of energy to protect women (and hence their babies) in times of famine. Not surprisingly, it's most resistant to dieting, and it makes so many women feel unattractive and miserable that a vast industry has blossomed around it offering all sorts of pseudoscientific treatments.

If only a diet existed that could get rid of cellulite without starving you to death. If only skilful massage could recontour the hips and thighs. If only special exercises could burn up the fat in your lower half. But the sad truth is that none of these things work. The only direct approach is liposuction, which involves sucking out some of the fat through a perforated tube or cannula inserted through one or more small incisions.

However difficult it can be to lose those obstinate inches from your hips and thighs, it's likely that losing weight will help to smooth away some of the cellulite so that you look and feel a whole lot better. And, anyway, what are a few dimples between friends?

dramatic results. The weight loss will be very slow, maybe only a pound or two (less than a kilo) a week. But it will be steady and, most important, it will be sustainable.

Why diets don't work in the long run

One of the big problems with dieting, quite apart from all that self-denial and straining of willpower, is the fact that our body chemistry is likely to respond to the shortage of calories by *conserving* body fat. If the diet is too strict, the metabolism adopts a kind of 'siege economy' as a natural response to famine. The metabolic rate slows down, burning fewer calories, and more of the calories in the body's system are diverted into fat stores as a defence against starvation, in effect 'locking in' body fat. This is why so many dieters find that, while they might lose a fair amount of weight to start with, they get to a point where they can't seem to shift any more. Their weight loss levels off.

This is a particular problem with diets that promise that you'll 'lose 7 pounds in 7 days' or offer similarly stunning results. These 'crash' diets are always very low in calories and most of the weight you will lose isn't fat – it's water. Yes, plain old common or garden H_2O, which is released when your starving metabolism burns up the most available stores of instant energy, the quick-release glycogen (body-starch) in your liver and muscles. Only when that's pretty well depleted do you start the much slower process of breaking down body fat – or not, as the case may be. More likely, you'll hit the dieters' plateau and struggle to lose any further weight at all. Worse still, if you ease up on the diet, your metabolism will build up its emergency glycogen stores again and you'll actually put on weight – the infamous yo-yo dieting.

The way to avoid this problem is to steer clear of any kind of crash diet or very low-calorie diet offering rapid results. If you take in enough calories to ensure that your metabolism doesn't re-adjust any of its settings and lock in your body fat, while consuming fewer calories than necessary to power all your activities, you will steadily lose weight. And that lost weight will be body fat that has been broken down slowly to provide the necessary fuel.

For the average adult, a daily calorie gap of 500 calories (where your food and drink provide 500 calories less than your body needs to stay the same weight) should result in a weight loss of about a pound a week. A gap of 1,000 calories should double that. To lose weight sensibly you should be aiming for a daily calorie gap of somewhere between those two amounts. But don't be tempted to aim for a gap any bigger than 1,000 calories or you'll trigger the dreaded lock-in of your body fat.

I don't want to confuse you. Remember, we're talking about the calorie deficit here – the difference between what you eat (your calorie intake) and what you need to maintain your current weight. For example, a woman of average height (5'4") with a sedentary lifestyle and two stones overweight requires about 2,000 calories a day to stay the same weight. A 500 calorie deficit (to lose about 1lb a week) would take that down to 1,500 calories a day, and a 1,000 daily deficit (to lose about 2lb) to just 1,000 calories a day. An average height man (5'9"), sedentary and two stones overweight, requires about 2,500 calories to maintain his current weight. A 500 calorie deficit will leave him with an intake of 2,000 calories, and a 1,000 calorie deficit drops it to 1,500 calories a day.

 The good news is that, by increasing the amount of exercise you take, you can increase the gap between calories expended and calories consumed without triggering the starvation mode.

The message is clear: to sustain your weight loss, slow and steady is the way. Slim by stealth. And to keep the weight down you need to be more active. See the 'Being more active' chapter.

Did you know? If a normal weight adult consumes just 60 calories (half a slice of bread) more than they expend in being active, they will be obese within 10 years.

Regular exercise stimulates your metabolic rate and meal-induced heat production (thermogenesis). You will burn more calories even while you sleep!

Tailoring your weight loss programme

Believe it or not, the more overweight you are, the less strict your diet should be. This is because heavier people have a higher metabolic rate (they burn more calories doing nothing) and severe restriction of calories is more likely to trigger their starvation mode. The chart below gives you an idea of the rate at which you should lost weight. If you stay within the middle band your progress will be sure and steady.

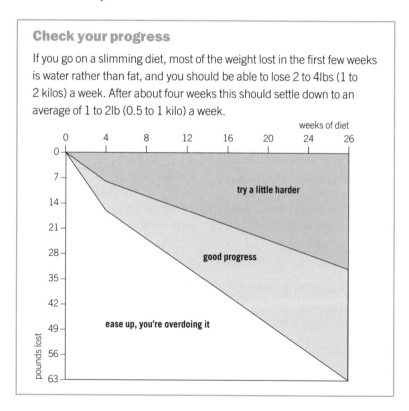

Check your progress

If you go on a slimming diet, most of the weight lost in the first few weeks is water rather than fat, and you should be able to lose 2 to 4lbs (1 to 2 kilos) a week. After about four weeks this should settle down to an average of 1 to 2lb (0.5 to 1 kilo) a week.

This is not a diet book and I haven't the space to go into details and give any sample diet plans. But calorie counters, which can be found in bookshops and supermarkets, will tell you what you can eat and drink within your daily allowance.

Remember a few basic rules. Even though you're reducing calories, always make sure you eat a healthy balanced diet, with plenty of fruit and vegetables and a moderate proportion of starchy staples like rice, potatoes and bread. Make sure you have three meals a day. The usual pattern is a light breakfast of cereal and fruit, a light sandwich or salad lunch and a more substantial two-course evening meal. Don't forget to include drinks in your calorie allowance. Every now and then give yourself a little treat. And keep yourself active. Think of the rewards – the more active you are, the more you can eat and drink!

Losing weight without counting calories

Please don't be put off by all this talk of calories. If you're someone who can't be fussed about calculating how many calories there are in this or that food, there's really no need to count them at all. All that's required is a rough idea of where the calories are in your food and drink – in other words, which things are more 'energy-dense' or, in plain-speak, more fattening. The short answer, of course, is anything that is high in fat, sugar or alcohol. See below for more information on where those calories are coming from.

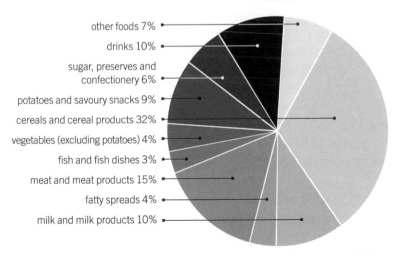

other foods 7%
drinks 10%
sugar, preserves and confectionery 6%
potatoes and savoury snacks 9%
cereals and cereal products 32%
vegetables (excluding potatoes) 4%
fish and fish dishes 3%
meat and meat products 15%
fatty spreads 4%
milk and milk products 10%

This chart shows the sources of calories in the UK diet.

Cut down on fat

Let's start with fat. Fat (including oil) is the most calorie-packed of all our nutrients. Every gram is loaded with 9 calories: that's about 40 calories per level teaspoonful (roughly the amount of butter or margarine you'd smear on your toast). So, where is the fat in your food?

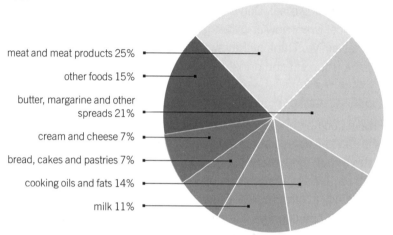

meat and meat products 25%

other foods 15%

butter, margarine and other spreads 21%

cream and cheese 7%

bread, cakes and pastries 7%

cooking oils and fats 14%

milk 11%

This chart shows the percentage of fat that comes from the different types of food that make up an average everyday diet.

By going easy on the major culprits you will be significantly cutting down on your calorie intake. Choosing leaner cuts of meat, removing visible fat, going easy on fatty meat products like sausages and pies, using a low-fat spread or spreading butter more thinly, avoiding fried foods, using skimmed or semi-skimmed milk, going for low-fat cheeses and so on are all small changes that can help to tip the balance in your favour. And you can always check the labels to see how much fat you're avoiding.

Go easy on the sugar

Next up is sugar. Sugar is about half as calorie-packed as fat – about 4.5 calories per gram. On average, we eat nearly a kilo of sugar a week, mostly without realising it. That's a large sackful in a year. Sugar is neat calories with virtually no other nutrient value at all, whether it's white, brown or any colour in between. We all know that we should be wary of sweets, cakes, biscuits, and sugary drinks. But what about all that 'hidden' sugar in our food – in breakfast cereals and savoury things like baked beans, sauces and prepared meals? Again, it's sensible to check the labels. Watch out for words like dextrose, sucrose, maltose, lactose, glucose, fructose or natural sweetener – they're all just sugar.

Watch the alcohol

And there's alcohol. If you drink two or three drinks (units) of alcohol a day, that could amount to 200 to 300 calories or about 10 per cent of your total daily calorie intake. Like sugar, alcohol is 'empty' calories with virtually no other nutrient value, although there is some evidence that moderate alcohol intake of one or two units a day can benefit the cardiovascular system and help to prevent a heart attack. Perfect excuse!

We talk much more about alcohol in 'Playing safe', but as a rough rule of thumb each unit of alcohol contains about 100 calories and one unit is equivalent to:

- one small glass of wine (not the bucket they give you in the wine bar)
- half a pint of ordinary strength beer, lager or cider (that's about 3.5 per cent alcohol by volume – not the premium 4 or 5 per cent stuff)
- one standard glass of sherry, port, madeira or other fortified wine
- one pub measure of spirits (vodka, gin, whisky, brandy, rum, etc)
- one shot of liqueur

But remember that 100 calories is just in the alcohol itself, not the whole drink. Needless to say, sweeter drinks, such as sweet or semi-sweet wines, sweet sherry, madeira, liqueurs or anything with a sugary mixer added (lemonade, bitter lemon, cola, tonic water, etc) will have quite a lot of extra calories on top.

Burning the calories – which activities are best?

There are two ways of tackling this question. The simple answer is any activity that makes you puffed. The more puffed you are, the more calories you burn. So, for example, walking uphill (or upstairs) burns more than walking on the flat and a brisk stride more than a gentle stroll. As you become fitter, of course, you'll be less short of breath, but you'll be doing the same work and still be burning calories at the same rate. So calorie burning gets easier as you get fitter, which is nice.

The other answer to the question is any mix of activities you enjoy doing, or that you can easily incorporate into your everyday life, and that burn more calories than you're used to. This is a more softly, softly approach to exercise for those who have a horror of the whole idea. And it stands a better chance of being sustained, week in week out, year in year out, which of course is what needs to happen if you want to keep your weight down.

There's increasing evidence that regular exercise will also stimulate your body's basal metabolic rate (the energy you expend doing nothing other than keeping your heart, brain and other organs going) and meal-induced heat production (thermogenesis), so that you burn more calories when you're at rest – even while you sleep!

There's lots of advice on this sort of thing in the first chapter of this book. And yes, of couse you're allowed to put your feet up while you read it.

What about medical treatment and surgery?

The natural, healthy eating and active lifestyle approach outlined above is very much along the lines recommended by NICE, the UK National Institute for Health and Clinical Excellence. But if someone has severe obesity with complications, such as high blood pressure, high blood cholesterol or type 2 diabetes, and has struggled in vain to lose weight through a supervised lifestyle programme,

NICE recommends that doctors consider a course of anti-obesity medication. It's only a temporary measure of course – and doesn't tackle the fundamental problem – but it can sometimes break the deadlock and increase a person's motivation to redouble their efforts.

In very severe cases, the answer might be to have surgery. Various types of stomach operation can be very effective in helping people lose a great deal of excess weight, with potentially life-saving benefits to their health. If you want to find out this option then contact your GP or call NHS Direct. However, it's important that you've tried other options before this one.

There are a number of organisations that exist to help people lose weight. Weight Wise is an independent website run by the British Dietetic Association, with unbiased, easy-to-follow hints and tips based on the latest evidence to help you manage your weight for good (www.bdaweightwise. com). Commercial organisations such as Weightwatchers (www.weightwatchers.co.uk) and Slimming World (www. slimmingworld.com) also help some people shed the pounds.

Small changes, big difference

I hope that by the end of this chapter you'll feel ready to tackle any weight issues you may have, even it it's for the umpteenth time. Don't forget the main message: this isn't about losing weight fast – it's about losing weight for good. This is a long-term, gentle project which could pay dividends in a year's time.

Why not make a note of your weight now, in the back of this book? Then look through the list overleaf and follow a few of the suggestions. If you stick to them you will see a real difference when you get back on the scales in a few months' time.

Feeling good!

✓ choose low-fat alternatives and leaner cuts of meat

✓ read labels: check for hidden fat and sugar

✓ remove visible fat from meat

✓ grill rather than fry

✓ cut down on added sugar or use artificial sweeteners

✓ cut down on alcohol and sugary drinks

✓ don't skip meals

✓ avoid snacking and grazing – if you must have something 'right now' make it a piece of fruit

✓ aim to lose an average of 1 to 2lb (0.5 to 1kilo) a week

✓ don't cut anything out completely

✓ be a little more active every day

Stressing Less

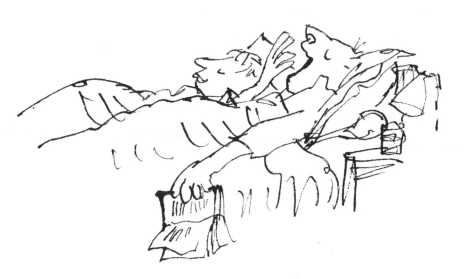

So far we've talked a lot about keeping active, eating a balanced diet and protecting ourselves from chronic ill-health. But what about knowing how and when to relax? For most of us, life is pretty hectic, and if we get the balance wrong, we suffer the consequences of stress. But what exactly is stress? What harm can it do? How can we avoid it? What are the best ways to relax? And how can we get a better night's sleep?

They say that one person's stress is another person's stimulus. Stress, whatever it is (there are literally dozens of definitions), is a natural part of life. Like temptation, stress is always with us, and always has been. The human race evolved with stress and we need some of the stuff in order to survive.

Way back in our hunter-gatherer days, stress was all around us. We were often in immediate danger – from warring tribes and hungry sabre-toothed tigers to disgruntled cavemates wielding clubs. So we evolved natural mechanisms to cope, referred to by scientists as the 'fight or flight response' but more commonly known as the 'instinct for survival'.

Not a great deal has changed. For many of us, life is still a struggle. We're still hunting and gathering – jobs, mates, possessions, bills. And there's no shortage of threats – relationship problems, money worries, job insecurity, fear of crime, terrorism, health concerns, bereavement. The warring tribes and sabre-toothed tigers haven't gone away.

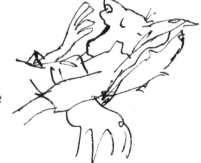

Stress or stimulus?

Stress is one of those fluffy words that mean different things to different people. We sometimes say we're suffering from stress, we're stressed out or we're under a lot of stress. But what exactly do we mean? It can range from pressure interfering with the way we relate to each other or do our everyday work to severe emotional problems and mental illness.

At its simplest, stress is a response to an immediate threat or tension – facing that sabre-toothed tiger or your dentist. Unless you have nerves of steel, the natural 'fight or flight' reaction kicks in: pounding heart, rapid breathing, tense muscles, jumpiness, tight chest, wide eyes, pallor and perhaps a cold sweat. This type of stress is usually over and done with fairly quickly. The tension or danger passes and your physiology returns to normal with no lasting ill-effects. All perfectly normal and healthy.

But, for some people, the tension becomes fear and the fear becomes panic. And, in some cases, just the anticipation of fear or embarrassment is enough to trigger the vortex of terror we call a panic attack (see page 105). This is a clear example of how a normal, healthy reaction to a stressful situation can be replaced by a crippling overreaction that then feeds on itself and becomes a long-term problem.

Of course, there's a thin line between terror and excitement. We all know people who become hooked on the adrenalin-fuelled high they get from extreme risk-taking, like bungee-jumping or running with the bulls in Pamplona. But many people suffer long-term psychological damage from a severe or repeated scare. An obvious example is survivors of a terrorist incident suffering post-traumatic stress disorder.

However, some of us thrive on the frisson of stress in our day-to-day lives. We prefer to work under pressure: deadlines, performance, risk. It challenges us and gives our lives a bit of edge. It plays to our thrill-seeking, competitive drive. It's not in the bungee-jumping league perhaps, but there's a welcome touch of adrenalin. People of this persuasion often approach retirement with some trepidation, thinking that without the stimulus of work they'll curl up in a ball and more or less cease to function. But more often than not, people like this find themselves as busy as ever, doing things they enjoy rather than chores imposed on them by others.

Chronic stress

Stress, as most people understand it, is not so much about being in frightening, competitive or challenging situations as about being subjected to relentless pressure, constant demands or repeated setbacks. It's a chronic, drawn-out state of affairs that grinds you down or works your nerves to a frazzle. A better word might be 'strain' because it can often feel like being stretched to breaking point or being put through the wringer and squeezed bone dry.

Good and bad stress

Good stress enables you to:	Bad stress can make you feel:
perform well	✘ ground down
face a crisis	✘ inadequate
meet deadlines	✘ powerless
compete with others	✘ frustrated
support friends and family	✘ trapped
take calculated risks	✘ strained
climb to the top of the heap	✘ isolated
work faster	✘ guilty
	✘ and utterly desperate

Causes of chronic stress are often intractable problems: a difficult close relationship (partner, child, neighbour, colleague, boss); a boring, repetitive job in which you have very little control or feel undervalued; no job at all, and no sign of one despite your best efforts; mounting debts you never seem to be able to get on top of; chronic ill-health that never gets any better; loss of your nearest and dearest; and generally any situation in which you feel there's no light at the end of the tunnel. It's this kind of stress – when it all gets too much, and you feel trapped, inadequate, guilty or ground-down, and basically can no longer cope – that is most likely to cause stress-related health problems.

Life event stress scale

life event	stress score
death of spouse	100
divorce	73
marital separation	65
prison sentence	63
death of close family member	63
personal injury or illness	53
marriage	50
redundancy or dismissal	47
marital reconciliation	45
retirement	45
change in health of close family member	44
pregnancy	40
sexual difficulties	39
gaining a new family member	39
change in personal finances	38
mortgage difficulties	32
change in work responsibilities	29
change in living conditions	25
trouble with boss	23
change in working hours	20
change in social activities	17
going on holiday	13
spending Christmas alone	12

Based on a survey of nearly 400 adults by Holmes and Rahe, 1967. Participants were asked to score the various events according to how stressful they regarded them compared with the death of a spouse scoring 100.

Many of these issues loom large in middle age: the 'mid-life crisis', when we question who we really are, what we stand for and what we want to do with the rest of our lives; the 'empty nest syndrome', when the kids leave home and we are left with heartbreaking echoes of laughter and mayhem, bedrooms still crammed with childhood paraphernalia, and everything is much too tidy and quiet. Other major life changes include the menopause, when a woman's dwindling hormones can bring on so many changes, mostly unwelcome, and retirement, when we relish or dread a new chapter in our lives with more time and less money. Failing health, or at best a feeling that one's body or brain aren't what they used to be, inevitably plays a part. And, of course, bereavement at the loss of someone very dear to our heart.

> **Did you know?** More people see their doctor about stress-related conditions than about coughs and colds. It's the second largest cause of sick leave in the UK, and costs the economy an estimated £6 billion a year.

Something's gotta give: stress-related problems

What 'gives' will vary greatly from person to person. So many maladies can be linked to stress – either triggered by it or worsened by it. Virtually every system in the body can be thrown out of kilter by its insidious effects. Here's a typical pick 'n mix of common stress-related health problems:

tired all the time	headaches	constant colds	
rheumatic pains	forgetfulness		difficulty sleeping
always irritable		loss of appetite	loss of libido
eating too much comfort food		drinking too much	
loss of interest in one's appearance			
feeling that everything's pointless			no joy in anything

There are plenty of others. And most of the above can be caused by things other than stress, perhaps by some underlying physical illness. Indeed, GPs spend a sizeable chunk of their working lives juggling with blood tests, x-rays and scans, trying to find out whether this or that symptom or illness might or might not be linked to stress.

And then there are the 'proper' medical conditions brought on or exacerbated by chronic stress. High blood pressure is a classic example. Asthma is another. Susceptibility to infections is a third. Others include irritable bowel, migraine, peptic ulcer, colitis, heart disease and various skin conditions. There are also the problems linked to smoking, drinking, over-eating, sexual excess and drug misuse that are often linked to stress. We'll be taking a closer look at this last group in 'Playing safe'.

The final group of stress-related conditions comprises the psychological problems we call anxiety states and depressive disorders. These are covered in more detail below.

All in all, stress-related problems cause an awful lot of human suffering and add up to a huge burden on society. In its broadest sense, stress is reckoned to be the second largest cause of sick leave and costs the UK economy an estimated £6 billion a year.

Is life really becoming more stressful?

We often talk about the stresses of modern living. Crime and fear of crime. The threat of terrorism. Concerns about new killer bugs like MRSA and bird flu. And everyday stresses such as the demand for higher and higher performance scores at work, traffic jams and computer crashes. Or just too much information.

Stress is blamed for more and more problems in life, and a huge multimillion pound industry has grown up around stress management. Thousands of therapists, counsellors, masseuses, complementary practitioners, yoga teachers and herbalists, not to mention purveyors of smooth dark chocolate, are all falling over themselves in a mad scramble to help us handle stress.

Most experts without an axe to grind are of the opinion that life is actually no more stressful than it was, say, 20, 50 or 100 years ago. It's just that we're all much more 'stress aware' these days. The stress management industry, aided and abetted by the media, is constantly pushing the stress message, so much so that we're in danger of becoming a nation of stressophobics – developing a morbid fear of stress, medicalising it and forgetting that most stresses are simply part of life's rich tapestry, for better or worse. At least, that's what the stress sceptics say. But, as you can imagine, there's no shortage of other experts who beg to differ.

Coping with stress

How we cope with these trials depends very much on our basic temperament and resilience. This is determined partly by our genes and partly by early life experience, but also by such crucial support as our family, friends and faith.

Everybody's different

One way of picturing this is to think of each of us having a 'stress thermostat'. For some of us, it's set high and things have to be pretty dreadful for us to feel stressed – the cool, calm, phlegmatic type. For others it's set low and the slightest adversity can really get to us – the highly strung, short-fused, panicky type. But most of us are somewhere between these extremes, and our setting on any particular occasion might depend on all sorts of things, including how well we slept the previous night, how hungry we are, where we are in the menstrual cycle, whether or not we're in pain, and how long it is since we won anything in the National Lottery. In other words, what kind of mood we're in.

The way stress affects us may not always be a simple matter of how irritable, short-tempered or cucumber-cool we are. Often the people who have most stress-related problems are those who bottle up their emotions and seem to be coping well, albeit through gritted teeth, while the fiery types who rant and rave and blow their top often manage to go through life with remarkably few psychosomatic ills.

Not that I'm an advocate of ranting and raving as a way of coping with stress, fun though it may be. But there's no standard answer for everyone, no one-size-fits-all magic stress-buster technique. We each need to work out what best suits us and our situation.

Crisis – what crisis?

It's important to recognise those times when stress is really getting you down. That's the first positive step you can take. Sit down with a pen and paper and write a list of everything that's worrying you. The next step is to ask yourself a few fundamental questions to get things in perspective. Questions such as:

- Who or what really matters in my life? My family? My friends? My job? My hobbies? My health?
- How much time should I give to each of these priorities?
- How much time should I have to just do what I want to do, rather than respond to other people's demands?
- What do I really enjoy? How can I make more time for it?
- What can I drop or ask someone else to do?
- Can I say 'no' to any of these?
- Which problems or issues are really bugging me?
- Can I sort out just one problem for now?
- Who can I share it with? Who can I ask for help?

Of course there may be no easy answers – or too many that conflict with each other. Priorities? They're all priorities! Drop something? How can I let that person down? Tackle one problem? What about all the other problems?

But sometimes, just by standing back for a moment and contemplating these questions, you can find a way through the maelstrom and out into the calm blue waters beyond. A course of action emerges. It may not be perfect. It may not be without risks or drawbacks. But at least it's a way forward. And if you stick to it, without letting yourself be sidetracked or discouraged, you'll find that other things fall into place and your stress miraculously diminishes. Believe me, it really can work.

Looking again at the list of questions above, in many ways, the most important is probably the last one about sharing your problems. Being able to talk them over with someone you feel at ease with is often half the battle. For many people it's a caring partner. But it could be another member of your family, a close friend, a member of your faith community, your doctor, a counsellor, or whoever you feel most comfortable with and who can help you order your thoughts, see things in perspective, strike a balance and find a way forward.

 Make a date with yourself – time just for you. Put it in your diary and keep it. Turn off your mobile phone. Simply chill out – listen to music, contemplate the clouds, sit by a fountain or waterfall, read a good book, watch the world go by.

Instant stress-busters

Sorting out your life is all very well, but what about dealing with the million and one so-called minor irritations that get right under your skin every single day? Lost keys, long queues at the checkout, constantly engaged phones, another light bulb going, the bus that sails past your outstretched hand, the cancelled train, traffic jams, corkscrew not in its proper place, no clean socks – you know the sort of thing. Any of these classic frustrations can push your blood pressure up a notch or two. And by the end of a fraught day you can

What is a panic attack?

A panic attack is a dreadful mounting fear that feeds on itself. A sheer blind terror, with a pounding heart, rapid shallow breathing, pale skin, cold sweat and spinning head. Some sufferers get a tightness in their chest and may feel faint, although few actually pass out. A typical attack lasts several minutes before easing off. About one person in 30 suffers a panic attack at some time in their life, many more women than men.

what triggers an attack?

Usually, being in some crowded place – a shop, a bus queue, a social gathering – and feeling trapped, exposed or embarrassed. Most sufferers are rather tense or anxious for some reason beforehand. Attacks tend to come in spates, every few days for about 2 or 3 weeks. But they may be much less frequent and go on for months or years. There's no fixed pattern.

what's the basic cause?

In some cases, it's the premenstrual syndrome; in others, the menopause. And often it's general stress, anxiety or an obsessive or compulsive personality. Panic attacks usually fade away when life becomes less hectic. There's a link between attacks and agoraphobia – the fear of going out, especially to enclosed public places. But which comes first – the panic attacks or the agoraphobia – is often not clear.

what's the answer?

Because the fear is coming from within rather than from the trigger situation itself, you must learn how to confront and control it. This means building up confidence in your ability to overcome the fear. One way is to use deep breathing to keep yourself calm while you deliberately face increasingly difficult situations. Many sufferers need the help of a psychotherapist. You can find one either through your GP or privately.

For support with panic attacks, contact No Panic, an independent charity with a nationwide network of volunteer counsellors (telephone helpline 0808 808 0545 (10am to 10pm daily); www.nopanic.org.uk).

be in such a frazzle that you have difficulty switching off and getting a good night's sleep.

It's worth learning a few simple tricks to stop yourself from exploding. Not easy if you're the exploding type. Smiling beatifically, turning the other cheek and following the path of Zen may work for some people, but you might need one or two more direct ways of calming your nerves – a few instant stress-busters. On pages 115–116 we explain three simple techniques: deep breathing, serene contemplation and progressive relaxation. More tried and tested ways of relieving stress are given below.

Massage

Massage is a direct physical way of soothing tense muscles and easing away tender trigger points and nodules. It's wonderfully relaxing, releasing those wicked little knots of spasm, especially in muscles normally held pretty rigid or static for most of the day, such as those in the back of your head, neck, shoulders and down your spine. Foot massage can be a real treat too.

There are just two big snags with massage (three, if you count finding yourself in the wrong sort of massage parlour). The first is that you need someone else to do the massaging for you, although this is really a blessing because it means you can just lie there and think of Thailand. The second is that whoever does it has to know what they're doing. There are dozens of different types of massage, using a wide range of techniques, with or without a dollop of aromatic oil and a hefty chunk of holistic philosophy. But in the end it all comes down to the hands. The kneading and stroking has to be absolutely right – too heavy and it's painful, too light and it tickles. Both are totally counterproductive.

Further information on massage can be obtained from the General Council for Massage Therapy, which is a non-profit-making body comprising the major professional associations in massage therapy in the UK (telephone 0870 850 4452; www.gcmt.org.uk).

Meditation

There are various meditation methods, some wrapped in several layers of oriental mysticism, philosophy or religion. But the simplest technique doesn't need any of that paraphernalia – just somewhere quiet and comfortable to sit or lie down.

Close your eyes and do some deep breathing and progressive relaxation. After a few minutes, focus your concentration on a point in the middle of your forehead, as if you were looking at it from the inside of your skull. Imagine yourself staring intently at this point, with your eyes shut. Think of the point as a narrow tunnel. Now let the tunnel draw you into it. Let it suck you in at an accelerating pace. Let it pull all your bodily tension through it into the far distance.

Once you've tried this a few times, you'll probably get the hang of it and you'll be able to slip into the tunnel much more quickly and easily. All your attention and all your worries will be drawn in, and within minutes your mind will feel wonderfully uncluttered. Whenever you want to, you can open your eyes and snap out of it, feeling remarkably refreshed.

Basically, meditation is just a simple form of mental concentration, focusing on a single featureless concept, which dampens down distracting thoughts and sensations and creates a feeling of mental clarity which can be quite euphoric. No mysticism is required, although the Eastern ancients didn't hesitate to make full use of it in their rituals and disciplines.

 Ask at your local library for details of meditation classes near you.

Yoga

Yoga has not only become one of the most popular ways of relaxing, but has also helped many thousands of people to rethink their entire life plans.

Yoga, in the fullest meaning of the word, is a philosophical and practical union of spiritual, moral, mental and physical fulfilment through a series of prescribed disciplines. The practice began in India about 5,000 years ago, but it's only in the past few decades that it has really caught on in such a huge way in the West.

The most widely practised type of yoga in the UK is hatha yoga, a combination of 'asanas' (physical exercises and postures), 'pranayama' (breathing techniques) and meditation. Its aim is to provide a balanced and wholesome approach to achieving perfect physical and mental harmony and tranquillity. At its simplest, the emphasis is on balance, muscle control and gentle stretching – all excellent ways of relaxing. Whether or not you want to get into the more philosophical or transcendental aspects of yoga is completely up to you, but even a little light yoga now and then can make you feel fantastic.

Yoga classes are widely available, and can be adapted to suit older people and those with various disabilities. There's also a good choice of books and DVDs on the subject.

See page 44 for advice on using yoga as part of an exercise regime.

Further information can be obtained from the British Wheel of Yoga, which is the governing body for yoga in Great Britain. It has a network of qualified yoga teachers throughout the country (telephone 01529 306851; www.bwy.org.uk).

...and countless other ways to relax

Hobbies, hot baths, aromatherapy, sex, listening to music, chilling out with friends and family, gardening, helping out in your local community – there are a thousand and one ways of taking your mind off your everyday worries and pressures.

Paradoxical though it may seem, any form of rhythmic, repetitive, dynamic exercise can help banish stress and lift your mood. Walking, dancing, skipping, cycling and swimming are all excellent stress-busters – as long as you can make enough time for them without getting stressed about it!

And, of course, there's always the ultimate relaxation therapy – a good night's sleep.

Getting a good night's sleep

Most people find that, as they move into middle age and beyond, they don't sleep as well as they used to. Their sleeping is lighter and more easily disturbed by noise or discomfort, and they don't feel as refreshed in the morning as they did in their younger days (hangovers aside).

About one person in ten has difficulty sleeping, but amongst the over-fifties there are at least twice as many. Whether it's difficulty nodding off, fitful sleep of poor quality or early waking, it's still a form of insomnia. The result is likely to be daytime drowsiness, tetchiness, poor performance, strained relationships, difficulty coping, depression, increased stress and anxiety, and an increased risk of accidents.

What causes insomnia?

There may be all sorts of reasons for insomnia in older people. Women going through the menopause are particularly likely to have disturbed nights – boiling hot one minute, cold the next, frequently waking drenched in sweat. Men in their sixties begin to suffer from a night-time urge to empty their bladder, brought on by a gradually enlarging prostate gland. Other problems might include:

- worrying about family, work or money
- aches and pains
- snoring partner
- sleep apnoea
- catnapping during the day
- tea, coffee, cheese or alcohol late at night
- being jumpy about intruders

- excitement about *Strictly Come Dancing*

There's no shortage of things to lose sleep over. And sometimes it's simply worrying about not getting enough of it – sleep that is. An anxious state of mind stimulates the brain to become hyperactive and prevents it from switching off at night, so that thoughts go round and round, and you lie there churning the same things over and over in your mind. The trouble is that once a pattern for not sleeping becomes established, it can be extremely difficult to break out of it.

What can be done about it?

First, don't be too concerned about not getting your full 8 hours. Research shows that, as we age, our brain and body need less sleep – more like 6 hours or even less, as long as it's good quality stuff, which, of course, it often isn't.

Avoid the triggers

To improve the quality of your sleep, first make sure that you avoid the obvious pitfalls:

- **tea and coffee** The stimulant effects of caffeine last several hours, so choose decaf
- **cheese** Strong cheeses contain amines, which can be psychoactive. Blue cheeses, in particular, can stimulate vivid dreams, which may disturb sleep
- **alcohol** This replaces the normal sleep pattern with an artificial somnolence which wears off after a few hours. The chances are you'll find yourself tossing and turning at 3am, reliving the entire evening – especially the embarrassing bits
- **exercise** Important though this is as part of your daily routine, you should avoid strenuous exercise late in the evening because it has a stimulant effect
- **scary movies** For obvious reasons. horror, violence or anything with Arnold Schwarzenegger in it

Snoring

It may seem comical, but snoring is no laughing matter. It probably causes more marital disharmony than deciding which TV channel to watch. And quite apart from the damage to relationships, the snorts, whistles and difficulty breathing also disturb the sleep of the snorer. This leads to daytime drowsiness, which can cause accidents at work or on the road. In many cases, especially in older people, snoring is linked to sleep apnoea, when breathing stops completely for about half a minute, perhaps dozens of times during the night. This may eventually lead to high blood pressure and heart trouble.

Who's most likely to snore?

Surveys show that half of all adults snore at least occasionally, and up to a quarter do so regularly. Snoring is about four times more common in men than women, is about three times as common in fat people as in thin ones, and gets worse as you get older. Occasional snorers usually only snore if they lie on their back, while regular snorers snore in any position.

Why does it happen?

The sound comes from vibrations of the soft palate when air is breathed in and out through the mouth. Eight out of ten regular snorers have a stuffy nose, often because the partition wall within the nose is crooked. Smoking or being in a smoky atmosphere makes the nose even stuffier. Drinking is another likely cause – alcohol relaxes the throat and prevents the snorer from waking and changing position.

What's the cure?

Avoid smoky atmospheres and alcohol in the evenings and lose excess weight. Decongestant nose drops should not be used regularly because they make the stuffiness worse. Special plasters and devices are available to prop open the nostrils or lift the jaw at night – ask your pharmacist or check the web. In severe cases, a simple operation on the soft palate or nasal septum may do the trick.

 Further information and a range of products are available from the British Snoring and Sleep Apnoea Association (telephone helpline 01737 245638; www.britishsnoring. co.uk).

Get comfortable

You can also do your best to ensure that your bed is comfortable by getting a better mattress and a bed-frame that doesn't squeak and creak, using comfortable pillows and bedclothes, and tweaking the heating so that you're neither too hot nor too cold.

Establish a routine

Next, establish a regular routine – almost a ritual – to condition your brain into sleepy-time mode. Perhaps some smooth music, some undemanding reading, a good soak in a nice warm bath, maybe a warm milky drink – or all of these wonderfully relaxing things at more or less the same time.

Another important aspect of the routine is to keep to regular hours whenever possible. Again, this is all part of the conditioning. Your brain has a natural rhythm throughout the night (and also, incidentally, throughout the day). Its activity fluctuates in a cycle roughly every 90 minutes. At night it dips down into deep sleep and then rises up to a lighter 'active sleep' phase (known as REM sleep) in which you dream, before sinking back down again into deep sleep. This cycle repeats four or five times a night, the dream phases lasting longer each time until you finally wake up, either naturally during the last, longest and lightest dream phase or when the alarm cruelly drags you from somewhere deep in the Land of Nod.

By keeping to the same lights-out and wake-up time night after night (especially wake-up time), you should be able to train your brain to dip down effortlessly into deep sleep at the beginning of the night, and enjoy a satisfyingly long dream phase at the end, so that you wake up feeling refreshed and raring to go. This may mean using an alarm clock for at least a week or two while your brain gets attuned to the time for waking up. It also means that, if you're lying there wide awake in the middle of the night, you should resist the temptation to put the light on and read for a while, or to raid the fridge, because this will simply reinforce and perpetuate the abnormal pattern, turning it into chronic insomnia.

What about sleeping tablets?

Twenty years ago, sleeping tablets were the standard remedy for insomnia. But we now know what a generally bad idea they were, and these days they are not commonly prescribed. Possible problems with sleeping tablets include:

- dependence (addiction), with severe withdrawal symptoms
- daytime drowsiness, which could be dangerous if driving or operating machinery
- night-time confusion and unsteadiness, which could cause a fall
- tolerance, which could mean the need to prescribe higher and higher doses to have an effect

Doctors still do sometimes prescribe sleeping tablets but usually only for a short time to get over a particularly bad patch, such as a sudden bereavement.

 The sleep council is a non-profit-making organisation which provides helpful advice on how to improve sleep quality and on how to choose the right bed (telephone 01756 791089; www.sleepcouncil.org.uk).

Small changes, big difference

OK. Now you're so thoroughly relaxed you can hardly raise an arm to turn over the page. Well, perhaps not. None of us can really expect to cut stress out of our lives entirely, but you'll probably feel better knowing that many of us are in the same boat, and that there are a few things you can do to make your stress more manageable.

And remember that you can't change everything at once: a few small changes will have a big impact on the rest of your life and leave you feeling better able to cope. Why not pick just one of the following and do it straightaway?

Feeling good!

- ✓ decide what is most important in your life
- ✓ talk to someone about your problems
- ✓ book some quality time just for you
- ✓ learn to say no to work and yes to fun
- ✓ spend ten minutes a day meditating or doing simple exercises
- ✓ take a walk in the park
- ✓ write a fresh 'to do' list every day
- ✓ be realistic and give yourself more time to get things done

Three stress-busters

1 Deep breathing

When you're really tense, you take rapid shallow breaths through your mouth using the upper part of your chest. By controlling your breathing so that you inhale slowly and deeply through your nose, using your diaphragm, you can instantly ease away tension.

If possible, sit comfortably and shut your eyes. Start by taking in a very long steady breath right into the deepest corners of your lungs. Hold it for a few seconds and then let it out very slowly without forcing. Just let the air flow out under its own momentum.

With the next breath, don't deliberately breathe in, let it happen naturally, only as deeply as it wants to. Hold it a few seconds, and relax. The same again with the next breath. And again with the next. After a few breaths you'll notice that your chest is doing less and less of the work and your tummy more and more. Eventually, with each breath, your tummy bulges slightly and your chest doesn't move at all. This is deep abdominal breathing. Very relaxing. Works a treat in traffic jams.

2 Serene contemplation

In the same way that we can become tense and anxious just by imagining something scary, so we can help to calm ourselves by thinking about something soothing and tranquil. This is also known as guided imagery.

Make yourself as comfortable as possible and shut your eyes. Try to imagine yourself in a scene that conjures up a feeling of serenity – perhaps lying on a sun-drenched beach, listening to the waves gently lapping on the shore, or sitting on a mossy bank by a waterfall, or in your favourite place in the country with the birds singing and the wind in the trees, or enjoying a warm embrace with someone you love dearly. Wallow in the scene for as long as you can spare. Believe me, it's a revelation. Excellent for computer rage and sitting in the dentist's chair.

3 Progressive relaxation

Here's one that uses muscle relaxation to ease away tension. Again, if you can, sit comfortably with your eyes shut. Then clench your fists very tightly and hold them clenched for a few seconds. And relax. Next, hunch your shoulders, hold them hunched for a few seconds – and relax. Then screw your face into a tight wince, as if someone was about to pop a large balloon right in front of your nose. Hold for a few seconds – and relax. Finally, do all these manoeuvres at once. Hold. And then slowly relax everything, feeling the tension drain away. After you've done this a few times, you'll get quite adept at it. You'll find it particularly handy just before important interviews, presentations, speeches or meetings with the bank manager.

You can use any combination of these three for added effect, or take them to a higher level through meditation (see page 107).

Playing safe

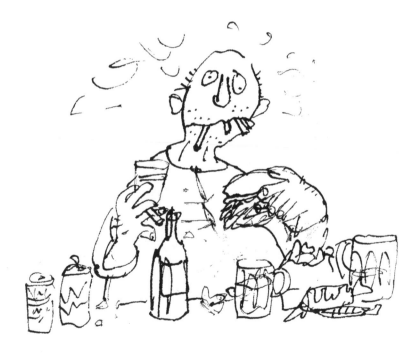

OK you're doing the right things. You're keeping yourself active, eating plenty of fruit and veg, watching your weight, finding great ways of relaxing and sleeping like a baby. All in all, you're well on the way to feeling fantastic. But, wait a moment. What about the many rocks on the road ahead? Life is full of health risks. How can you have lots of fun without paying the price?

This chapter will help you play safe by giving practical advice on:

- giving up smoking for good
- drinking without tears
- enjoying sex safely
- holidaying well

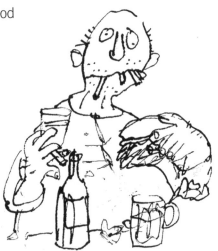

Smoking: how to give up for good

We all know how unhealthy smoking is. Taking the hit are your lungs (chronic bronchitis and cancer), heart (angina and heart attack), blood vessels (high blood pressure and gangrene), nasal passages (sleep apnoea), throat (cancer) and, rather surprisingly, bladder (smoke toxins are concentrated in the urine and can cause cancer).

Most smokers would like to pack it in but fail to get over the nicotine withdrawal period, which can be quite a struggle. After all, nicotine is as addictive as heroin and giving up is not always that easy. So, just in case you're one of them, here are my Five Steps to Successful Stopping.

Step 1 Convince yourself

As with breaking any habit, to succeed you have to be really committed to the idea. No one can make you give up. You are the one in charge. You have to convince yourself that you would rather be a non-smoker, and that you want to be one right now. A good starting point is to remind yourself why giving up is such a good idea.

Be a whole lot healthier

Within hours of giving up, your body expels carbon monoxide and many other poisons inhaled in cigarette smoke. Within days, your breath will be fresher, your teeth cleaner and your breathing easier. Within a few weeks you'll feel fitter. Within months, your risk of heart problems will start to diminish and the self-cleaning mechanism will help your lungs recover. You may be getting on in life, but there's still much to be gained by stopping smoking right now (see page 120).

Feel clean and fight pollution

No longer will you taint the air around you, your hair, your clothes, your car, your home. No longer will you have to sneak outside for a quick one or spray the place with air-freshener.

The big gains from giving up

Within 20 minutes your blood pressure and pulse rate should return to normal.

Within 8 hours oxygen levels in your blood should return to normal. Carbon monoxide is halved, nicotine is down by a quarter.

Within 24 hours all carbon monoxide has been eliminated from your body. Your lungs start to clear out mucus and other smoking debris.

Within 48 hours there is no nicotine left in your body. Your ability to taste and smell may be greatly improved.

Within 72 hours breathing becomes easier. Your bronchial tubes begin to relax and your energy levels increase.

In 2 to 12 weeks circulation improves throughout the body.

In 3 to 9 months coughs, wheezing and breathing problems get better as your lung function is increased by up to 10 per cent.

In 1 year the risk of a heart attack drops to about half that of a smoker.

In 10 years the risk of lung cancer falls to half that of a smoker.

In 15 years the risk of heart attack falls to the same as someone who has never smoked.

Save money

Work out how much you'll save each month by not smoking. This becomes even more of an issue when you're on a pension.

Step 2 Make the decision and stick to it

Having convinced yourself that you want to stop smoking, now make a firm decision to do so. Don't keep putting it off, waiting for the perfect time. Don't vacillate, unsure of whether you'll succeed this time or whether it's worth going through that denial all over again only to cave in at the end. Tell yourself that you can do it, and that you will do it. This time it's for real. And mean what you say. Make a pledge to yourself or your partner or friend.

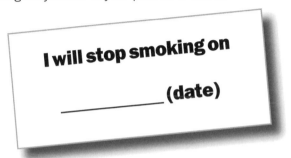

I will stop smoking on
_____ (date)

Step 3 Prepare to stop

As with any battle, preparation is vital. Make a firm date to give up within the next fortnight. Put it in your diary and tell everyone. You may need their encouragement and support. If you can persuade your partner or a friend to give up with you, so much the better. In the week before Stop Day, cut down the number of cigarettes you smoke – miss out the less important ones. One trick is to put a rubber band round the packet so you have to ask yourself each time, 'Do I really need this one right now?' Another trick is to not carry a lighter so you have to keep asking for a light. If you're very dependent on smoking you should consider anti-smoking medication or nicotine replacement treatment from your GP or pharmacist.

Step 4 Stop Day

The moment you wake up, tell yourself you are now a non-smoker. Make this crucial mental leap. Instead of thinking of yourself as a smoker trying to give up, you are now a non-smoker who doesn't do cigarettes. You don't need them. You can manage perfectly well without them. You will go through the whole of today without putting a cigarette to your lips. You don't smoke because you're now a non-smoker. Practise saying, 'No thanks, I don't smoke' over and over again.

Don't worry about tomorrow. Just make sure that you get through this first day without a cigarette. Help yourself by removing all cigarettes, lighters, ashtrays and other smoking accoutrements from your environment, including secret hiding places. Carefully avoid trigger situations. For example, drink orange juice instead of coffee, have a sandwich in the park instead of a pub lunch, chew sugar-free gum when you're on the phone. Find diversions and distractions to take your mind off fags. If you get a strong craving, try deep breathing (see page 115) or phone a friend to talk you out of it.

Step 5 Stay stopped

Follow the same principles as for yesterday. Just take one day at a time, and aim to get through each day without a fag. Find non-fattening things to chew or munch, things to do with your hands, fresh-tasting drinks instead of coffee or tea, new places to go in your breaks.

No thanks – I don't smoke

If you're worried about putting on weight, surround yourself with low-calorie comforters: mineral water, low-cal drinks, sugar-free gum, pieces of fruit.

Keep on your guard. It's very tempting after a week or two – or a few months – to convince yourself that you've cracked it and that it won't do any harm to allow yourself one little ciggie as a reward. Classic error! Remember you're a non-smoker. You don't smoke any more.

Never be tempted to have just one little ciggie or even a drag. There is no such thing as just one. The first puff heralds the end of your life as a non-smoker.

The craving will only last a short time, so tell yourself to hold out just a bit longer; if you can resist the urge for five minutes it will pass – and you'll feel so proud of yourself.

Find support

You might find it easier, particularly if you're a heavy smoker, to give up with the support of your GP, practice nurse or pharmacist through your local NHS Stop Smoking Service. This provides anti-smoking medication, including nicotine gum or patches, on prescription (free for people who don't pay prescription charges). Recent research has shown that a smoker who tries to quit with the NHS Stop Smoking Service is up to four times as likely to succeed than by willpower alone.

Nicotine replacement products are also available without prescription over the counter at pharmacists. There are also some excellent books and websites on giving up smoking, and hypnosis or acupuncture can certainly help some people to succeed.

You can find out more about local services, including one-to-one counselling and stop smoking groups, by phoning the NHS Smoking Helpline or visiting the website. Both individual and group sessions provide helpful information and practical advice, such as tips on beating cravings, choosing the right day to give up, and how to get medication such as bupropion on prescription. Many people find that joining a group provides extra encouragement to quit.

For help with giving up smoking, contact the NHS Smoking Helpline (telephone 0800 169 0 169; www. gosmokefree.co.uk). QUIT is an independent charity whose aim is to save lives by helping smokers to stop, with a particular emphasis on nicotine replacement (telephone helpline 0800 00 22 00; www.quit.org.uk).

Drinking without tears

Most of us get a great deal of pleasure from a glass or two of fine wine, a pint of real ale or that early evening gin and tonic. Indeed, for some of us, life wouldn't be the same without it. And we all know how a roomful of rather shy and reserved people making polite conversation about pruning roses or the traffic on the A36 can become a riot of laughter and camaraderie after a few top-ups. So how can nature be so perverse, giving us all the joys of alcohol with one hand and all the horrors with the other?

> **Did you know?** The parts of your body that take the hit from alcohol are mainly your liver and brain, although your stomach, pancreas, ovaries and testicles may also suffer.

Alcohol and your liver

Most of the work of dealing with alcohol in the system is done by the liver, the body's main chemical factory and detoxification plant. Some alcohol is breathed out, peed out or sweated out, but the liver bears the brunt. Despite its potential benefits in small doses, alcohol is basically a toxin. It damages cells and, in doing its selfless detox work, the liver is directly in harm's way. The liver cells respond at first by becoming filled with a fatty substance rather like foie gras. Heavy binges may be followed by inflammation of the cells. And if the excess drinking continues over a period of years, the consequence is likely to be scarring of the liver – the process we call cirrhosis.

Cirrhosis used to be mainly a disease of people in their fifties and sixties (they rarely survived into their seventies), but we're now in the throes of an epidemic of alcoholic liver disease (a doubling of cirrhosis over the past decade). And more and more cases are now occurring among 30- and 40-somethings.

At moderate levels of drinking, the liver can cope with the insult and recover quickly. Indeed, it gets rather used to the business of breaking down alcohol. But once drinking gets above the sensible limits and into the danger zone, problems begin. Women's livers are far more susceptible to alcohol than men's, and a large glass of wine at lunchtime and two more in the evening could, over a period of years, cause hepatitis and liver damage. Also, as we get older, we are all less able to tolerate alcohol. So, once again, it's all too easy to slip into a habit that is harmful to health without having an obvious drinking problem.

Alcohol and your brain

There's no doubt that alcohol consumed in large quantities kills neurones stone dead, and this lost grey matter can never be replaced. Heavy drinkers have shrunken brains and lose much of their ability to think clearly and remember things. But what does moderate drinking – one or two units a day – do to your brain?

Well, the good news is that most scientific studies so far seem to suggest that it may actually help to prevent the deterioration in short-term memory, quick thinking and spatial awareness that so often accompanies the ageing process. Doctors following up thousands of middle-aged people over many years have tended to find a positive association between moderate alcohol intake and cognitive ability. This isn't conclusive – the evidence is still coming in – but, yes, that daily tot may truly be a tonic in more ways than one.

Alcohol and your heart

The other good news about alcohol is its potential benefits for the heart and circulation. There's now strong evidence that drinking one or two units a day is associated with a lower risk of coronary heart disease, whether you're male or female, under or over 65. This holds true even after allowing for other risk factors such as smoking, exercise, diet, blood pressure and the like. The reduction in risk can be anything up to 50 per cent, but it takes several years for this to show itself. Incidentally, it doesn't matter whether you're drinking red wine, white wine, beer, spirits or Harvey Wallbangers because the active ingredient is the alcohol itself, and it seems to work by raising the level of HDL cholesterol ('good' cholesterol) in the bloodstream.

Before you stock up your medicines cupboard with your favourite tipple, please note that the British Heart Foundation does not recommend that we take up daily drinking to stave off heart disease. They point out that there's a fine line between benefit and risk with alcohol, and we should focus our efforts on the healthier options of stopping smoking, eating a healthier diet and taking more exercise.

Alcohol and blood pressure

While one or two units of alcohol a day might be beneficial for the heart and circulation, regular drinking of three or more could start to push up your blood pressure. And the more you drink above the recommended sensible limit, the greater your risk of hypertension. Heavy drinkers treble the odds against themselves and are lining up for the consequences of uncontrolled high blood pressure – a stroke, heart attack or chronic kidney disease. What's more, in many cases, the alcohol interferes with the medication, making effective control of blood pressure particularly difficult.

Is it true that red wine is better for you than white?

There does seem to be increasing evidence that red wines contain more antioxidants than white wines, and that they may have an additional heart-protecting effect if consumed in moderation (no more than a small glass or two a day). UK scientists have found that the more tannic red wines – such as those from south-west France, which are fermented for longer with the grape skins and pips – seem to have the most potent protective effect on the inner lining of the arteries. Interestingly, the inhabitants of south-west France are noted for their longevity. But this could be for any number of reasons, not least of which is their high consumption of fresh fruit and vegetables, loaded with – you guessed it – antioxidants.

Alcohol and accidents

One or two small glasses of wine might be good for the long-term health of your brain or heart, but by golly they can play havoc with your ability to drive, mow the lawn, climb a stepladder or bang a nail in a wall. Just one drink can double your risk of an accident, and two in quick succession can multiply it fourfold. The horrifying fact is that anyone who is just below the UK legal limit for driving (blood-alcohol level 80mg/100ml) is up to ten times more likely to crash or cause an injury than if they hadn't had a drink. No wonder there is mounting pressure on the government to bring the limit down to 50mg/100ml in line with a number of other countries in Europe.

Basically it takes less alcohol than you might think to push you over the legal limit. How many drinks will depend on a whole range of factors: how tall you are, how plump, what's in your stomach, how quickly you've been drinking, when you had your last drink, how much alcohol was in it, and so on. The most sensible thing is not to have any alcohol at all if you're driving.

Incidentally, a lot of people think a strong cup of coffee is a good antidote. It isn't. You just have to wait until the alcohol leaves your system at the rate of about one unit per hour. Perhaps the most sobering thing is to remember the penalties – a hefty fine and surrendering your licence.

Oh, and back to the subject of stepladders. Alcohol is implicated in a third of all domestic accidents. So don't think you're entirely safe even if you stay at home.

How much is too much?

Here's what the Department of Health says ... you have been warned!

Men Not more than 3 or 4 units in 24 hours.
Consistent drinking of 4 or more units a day is not advised.

Women Not more than 2 or 3 units in 24 hours.
Consistent drinking of 3 or more units a day is not advised.

How many units in your glass?

Until they standardise the labelling, it's difficult to know quite how much alcohol you're drinking. Here's a quick run down of the number of units* in typical drinks:

large 250 ml glass of red or white wine (13 per cent)	3.3 units
pint of best bitter (5.2 per cent)	3 units
pint of strong lager (5.2 per cent)	3 units
pint of strong cider (5.3 per cent)	3 units
standard 175 ml glass of red or white wine (13 per cent)	2.3 units
pint of ordinary strength bitter (4 per cent	2.3 units
pint of ordinary strength lager (4 per cent)	2.3 units
pint of stout (4 per cent)	2.3 units
double measure (50 ml) of standard strength liqueur	2 units
small 125 ml glass of red or white wine (13 per cent)	1.6 units
275 ml bottled alcopop	1.4 units
single 25 ml measure of spirits (gin, vodka, rum, whisky, brandy)	1 unit
standard glass of sherry, port, martini etc	0.9 units

*1 unit = 10ml of pure alcohol

Is your drinking becoming a problem?

It may not always be obvious to you or others that you have a drink problem. Here are ten questions to ask yourself.

- Do you ever lose time from work due to drinking?
- Does your drinking ever upset your home life?
- Do you sometimes feel guilty or regretful about your drinking?
- Do you ever want a drink in the morning?
- Does drinking interfere with your sleep?
- Do you drink to escape from worries or trouble?
- Do you often drink alone?
- Do you drink to build self-confidence?
- Have you ever experienced a loss of memory through drinking?
- Have you ever been to hospital for something linked to drinking?

If you answered yes to three or more of these, you probably have a drinking problem and should seek help sooner rather than later. Try to cut down and to have at least 2 alcohol-free days a week. Of course, this may be easier said than done, but there are lots of self-help books, leaflets and websites that offer help and advice about how you can stop or reduce drinking.

If you want to reduce your drinking, Drinkaware, run by an alliance between the drinks industry and government, is a friendly practical website with lots of helpful tips (www. drinkaware.co.uk). The charity Alcohol Concern has an online service to help you work out if you're drinking too much and a *Down your drink* programme which sets targets for cutting down. Its website lists other alcohol support services (www.alcoholconcern.org.uk). You can also call Drinkline, a confidential service offering help and support 24 hours a day, 7 days a week (telephone 0800 917 8282).

Talking sex

They say youth is wasted on the young. So perhaps is sex, although I don't recall wasting too much of it at the time. Youth may have more strength, suppleness and stamina but, hey, there's so much more to good sex than the three Ss. What youth lacks and we oldies have in abundance is the fourth S – subtlety. Sweet, sweet subtlety! In the eyes, the mouth, a smile, a word, a touch, a caress. In togetherness.

Sex in our fifties and above may not be as rampant as it was in our twenties and thirties. But that doesn't necessarily make it any the less enjoyable or satisfying. (I say 'necessarily' because you might disagree.) Sex isn't really about mechanics and dynamics and thrust and counterthrust. It doesn't conform to Newtonian principles. It's not about physics; it's about chemistry.

Right now, there's an ongoing debate about the joys of sex for the middle-aged woman. Fifty is the new 35 say the protagonists of 'great mature sex', fuelled by hormone replacement therapy (HRT), cosmetic surgery, Viagra, royal jelly, vaginal lubricants, vibrators and any number of other erotic additives and accoutrements. It's a time of liberation, they say – the kids have left the nest, contraception is irrelevant, the job is less onerous, perhaps there's a new relationship. 'What are you talking about?' says the opposition, who just can't see the joy in it, or just can't see it at all.

And what of mere men? Are we blokes engaging in this brouhaha? After all, we're rockers at heart aren't we? Forever feral. Always searching for the thrills of yesteryear? Well not necessarily. (I say 'necessarily' because you might disagree.)

Anyway, enough of idle speculation. Let's get down to brass tacks.

Sex and the older woman

Around the age of 50 is the time when a woman has to come to terms with the reality of no longer being fertile (although contraception should be continued for one full year after the last period or bleeding). Of course there's much more to the fifties than the menopause, but for some women it can certainly dominate proceedings. The symptoms, such as hot flushes, night sweats, depression and vaginal dryness, can play havoc with a woman's sex life and can drag on for many months or even years. HRT may solve many of these problems, and a vaginal gel lubricant or steroid-containing vaginal cream can greatly help relieve painful sex. But there's a downside to HRT. For more on the menopause, see page 171.

In emotional terms, women can sometimes lose confidence during the menopause. It's important not to give in to this. You've got years of health and happiness before you, and should look after yourself and take pride in your appearance.

Sex and the older man

For a man, there may be problems maintaining an erection (about 10 per cent of men in their fifties) and this too may strain a relationship. Most worries about libido stem from a media-driven ideal, an anxiety about what's expected or a yearning for lost youth. Both are false gods and are all too likely to end in disappointment, embarrassment, anxiety … and lost libido. More and more men are being prescribed Viagra or an equivalent to boost their sex drive and potency. (Recent evidence suggests that women, too, have a similar problem with their clitoris, although they may not realise it, and that stimulant medication such as Viagra may help them too.)

Nevertheless, according to researchers in Norway, men in their fifties are generally more satisfied with their sex lives than men in their thirties and forties. But, from 60 onwards, sexual satisfaction as such takes a plunge. Advancing age tends to be associated with a declining sex drive and ability to have an erection and ejaculate, although not so much with loss of pleasure. In other words, sexual function may diminish, but not necessarily sexual enjoyment. About 20 per cent of men in this age group have erectile dysfunction, but couples are much less likely to be bothered by it. Physical sex tends to be less frequent and less energetic in one's sixties. But cuddling and caressing can continue as much, if not more. The joy of older sex is no less fond, just less frenetic.

Sex and health

The primary concern when we're older tends to be our general health, physical and mental, which may affect our sex life. We do tend to have more aches and pains – perhaps the beginnings of arthritis or the back playing up. There may be more serious problems such as high blood pressure, diabetes or heart disease. Or anxiety and depression. Here are eight ways in which physical ill-health can spoil our fun.

Prescribed medication

Many common drugs are passion-killers. Pills for blood pressure, depression and heart trouble are the usual culprits. But there are usually alternative prescriptions for these conditions that don't have these side-effects. Check with your doctor.

Cardiac concerns

People who have had a heart attack or angina or have an irregular heartbeat are often worried that sex will finish them off. Out with a bang. But evidence suggests that, with modern treatment and a sensible rehabilitation programme, there's no reason why people with a cardiac history can't enjoy sex just as much as before. Ask your doctor about this.

Depression

This is certainly a downer, no question. Either the depression itself or its treatment. But once a person's mood has been lifted, so that talking treatments can be used and medication reduced, libido can make a comeback. See page 154.

Alcohol

Sex and alcohol are often good bedfellows – a great way to relax and let loose those inhibitions. But remember the old adage about alcohol provoking the desire and diminishing the performance. There's a fine line to be trodden. Too much alcohol can take the edge off things. More on page 123.

Sexually transmitted diseases

Just because you're over 50 doesn't mean that you're immune from all the sexual infections that are flying around. Chlamydia, gonorrhoea, herpes, genital warts, HIV – they are all as keen to invade your body as anyone else's. Unless you're with a trusted partner, always use a condom. This needn't interfere with sexual pleasure – indeed it can help you relax.

Stress

Busy high-pressure job, family crises, money worries, what colour to paint the kitchen – they can all take their toll on your sex life. It needn't be so. See the wise words about stress in 'Stressing less'.

Menopause

Mentioned above and elsewhere. There are many ways to minimise the negatives and take advantage of the positives. Not having to worry about contraception is a big plus.

Low self-esteem

Lacking confidence? Looking and feeling a mess? Hating yourself? Time to take charge and go for that makeover. New look. New hairdo. New way of life.

We can help fend off many of these problems by keeping active. This is the best way of giving ourselves a strong sense of well-being and physicality that improves sexual feelings. Many a flagging middle-aged sex life has been re-sprung through a regular programme of visits to the local leisure centre or frequent walks in the park or countryside, especially as a twosome.

 For more information on sexual health issues, contact the fpa, which offers high quality information and services for people throughout the country, regardless of sexual orientation (telephone helpline 0845 122 8690; www.fpa. org.uk).

Going places

For many of us, mid-life is our big chance to go places. Freed from the shackles of family and job, we can at last stretch our wings and see the world. And what a tonic travel can be. The excitement of the new – and the old. Exotic cultures, ancient civilisations, amazing vistas. A world of difference to be discovered out there waiting for us.

But (there's always a 'but' in health books) travelling has its pitfalls as well as its pleasures. The holiday of a lifetime can be ruined by some simple omission or mistake. Something so easily avoidable had you taken the right precautions.

Things to think about before you go

There are just a few things that might be needed by way of preparation – most of them injected into your left arm. Apart from jabs, you should take a supply of any regular medication you might be on, perhaps a few items by way of first aid and, if you're susceptible to it, motion sickness pills.

Travel jabs

Vaccinations are a pain. Not only the jabs themselves, but also the business of sorting out which ones you need and where to get them from. You can't help wondering whether they're absolutely necessary and whether maybe you could give them a miss.

But skipping your jabs is like playing Russian roulette. OK, you may be staying in a four-star hotel in Turkey or Goa. But how can you be sure that you won't come into contact with the germs that cause hepatitis or polio, meningitis or typhoid?

If you're travelling anywhere outside northern and western Europe, North America, Australia and New Zealand, you'll need the extra protection. But remember, there are all sorts of ifs and buts about each of these jabs, with different advice for people with certain allergies or anyone whose immune system is suppressed by steroids or HIV. So make sure you mention anything that might be relevant to your doctor or travel clinic beforehand.

What jabs for where?

It depends where you're going. Each country has its own range of commonly catchable diseases. Your travel company should be able to provide you with a list of recommended jabs. If not, ask your doctor or contact NHS Direct (telephone: 0845 4647), or you can check out the Department of Health website at www.dh.gov.uk (look for Health Advice for Travellers). The usual jabs for countries where standards of hygiene and sanitation are less than ideal are hepatitis A and typhoid. Others include polio (given by mouth, not injection), hepatitis B and C, meningitis, tetanus, diphtheria and rabies.

If you were born in the UK, you will probably have some immunity against some of these – polio, diphtheria and tetanus, for example – thanks to the jabs you had as a baby. But the chances are you'll need a booster dose for both polio and tetanus.

In most cases, these precautions are recommended, not compulsory. But you'd be taking a real chance if you went without them. Diseases can be picked up so easily – the ice in your cola, a mouthful of seawater, a cut foot, even a handshake.

For some countries, certain vaccinations are compulsory. For example, if you're going to any part of central America or central Africa, where yellow fever is rife, you'll need a yellow fever jab. What's more you'll need an international vaccination certificate as proof of vaccination in order to enter most other countries afterwards.

When and where should they be done?

Ideally, about 6 weeks before arriving at your destination to allow for the spacing of different jabs and doses. But certainly no less than 2 weeks, otherwise your immunity level won't have had time to build up.

Your own GP should be able to provide the basic ones, such as hepatitis A, typhoid and a tetanus or polio booster. You will probably have to pay a fee for this additional service, depending on the types of vaccination and number of doses needed. A certificate usually costs £10 to £15 extra.

If you need to go elsewhere for your jabs, a number of private companies run travel clinics. For example, MASTA and BUPA have clinics up and down the country. Look them up in your yellow phonebook. Again, fees vary considerably – but it's certainly not cheap.

As with any jab, you can expect some soreness where the needle went in, and maybe a slight feeling of listlessness. Some vaccinations can make you feel quite 'fluey', especially if you have several doses together or close to each other. A couple of paracetamols every 4 hours will usually be enough to tide you over. If you have a more severe reaction, see your doctor.

Malaria

Malaria is a potentially life-threatening fever caused by a tiny parasite caught from a single bite by an infected mosquito. It's a major problem in most tropical and some subtropical areas, although less so in big cities and on higher ground.

There is currently no vaccine against malaria. But if you're going to a malarial area, even just a stopover, you'll need to take a course of anti-malaria medication. There are several types, so ask your doctor or travel clinic about the pros and cons. The most important thing is to start the course at least a week before reaching the malarial area and continue it until a month after returning. While there, you should use plenty of insect repellent, keep your arms and legs covered after sunset and sleep under a mosquito net.

Travel health advice is available from Medical Advisory Services for Travellers Abroad (MASTA) through an online health brief and a network of travel clinics across the UK (www.masta.org). The Department of Health provides health advice for travellers at www.dhgov.uk.

Your medical bag

Prescribed medication First and foremost, if you're on regular medication – maybe for asthma, blood pressure, diabetes, a heart condition, epilepsy, or whatever – do make sure you take enough to cover your entire trip. You might also need either a letter from your doctor or a clinic note detailing your medication. Any medicines you take should be in their properly labelled containers.

First aid and prevention Insect repellent (look for one containing DEET), antiseptic cream, plasters, antidiarrhoea tablets and water sterilisation tablets won't take up much space and could be extremely useful. Many high street pharmacies sell basic first aid or medical kits with bandages, scissors and perhaps even sterilised medical equipment such as syringes, needles and suture materials.

Health insurance

This is essential. Make sure the level of cover is adequate – always read the small print and perhaps check with your travel company before you leave.

You should always take your European Health Insurance card EHIC) with you on visits to Europe. However, the EU reciprocal arrangement doesn't cover the costs of bringing a person back to the UK if necessary.

Dental care

If your teeth or gums are likely to need attention while you're away, try to visit your dentist before you leave. Dental treatment abroad is often difficult to find, of variable quality and may be very expensive.

Condoms

If you are not excluding the possibility of a sexual encounter with someone new, take condoms with you. They may not be readily available or of an adequate standard at your destination.

Reducing the risk of thrombosis

Deep vein thrombosis, or DVT, is a blood clot in one of the body's deep veins, usually in a leg. It's often caused by having to sit still for a long time, and the classic risk situation is travelling for long periods in a plane, train or car. Although it's fairly rare, older people are at increased risk. You can help to reduce that risk by taking a couple of aspirins at the beginning of your journey and doing simple exercises like flapping your feet and rotating your ankles. Better still, get up and walk around if you can and stay hydrated with regular non-alcoholic drinks.

Avoiding travel sickness

If you're travelling by sea but, like me, have trouble coping with anything more gastrically challenging than a dead flat calm, it might be sensible to take tablets for motion sickness. Ask your pharmacist for a formulation that doesn't make you drowsy. This is particularly important for drivers using the cross-channel ferry. Driving on the right is difficult enough when you're wide awake.

Things to do while you're there

Avoiding tummy troubles

Delhi belly, gippy tummy, Turkey trots, Montezuma's revenge. Lots of names for more or less the same thing. Misery. Even the smartest resorts can play havoc with your insides if you're not careful. And that fantastic brand new hotel on a stretch of unspoilt tropical shore is probably the worst. Stunning setting. Dreadful plumbing.

Most hot places (and quite a few not-so-hot places) are a health hazard as far as food and drink are concerned. Here are some basic tips to help steer clear of most nasties.

- Avoid drinking tap water, even in the plushest places. You really do need to be doubly sure that it's OK before you let it pass your lips, even just to brush your teeth.

- Always wash fruit and anything else that's going in your mouth, including your hands, in bottled water if necessary.

- Peel fruit before you eat it. But don't eat fruit that has been peeled for you, especially if it has been sitting around for a while.

- Beware of home made ice cream and lollies from street vendors or market stalls. Stick to branded ices.

- Avoid local cheeses, especially if you're pregnant (unlikely, I know). They may be contaminated with listeria or salmonella.

- If you're not sure about an eating place, don't be tempted by any meat, poultry, fish or shellfish dish unless it's properly cooked and served piping hot.

- If you do get the trots, drink plenty of bottled water or fruit juice, adding half a teaspoon of salt per litre to replace losses.

Safe in the sun

It seems a cruel irony that something as life-enhancing as sunshine should also be a source of potential danger. Basking near-naked in the warm sun is a pleasure for millions. But, as granny always said, you can have too much of a good thing, and those ultraviolet rays can work wicked tricks on the human skin given half a chance.

In small doses, sunlight is beneficial. Apart from bestowing warmth, the rays work on a substance within the deeper layers of the skin to produce a form of vitamin D. For many people on meagre diets in the developing world this is their only source of this important vitamin. However, the same rays that can boost health can also damage our skin in two fundamental ways: by destroying collagen, the protein that gives our skin its youthful elasticity, and by damaging DNA, the consequence of which is various types of skin cancer.

UV rays – the dangers Ultraviolet (UV) rays are actually invisible, but they have the power to penetrate skin and cause mischief by:

- causing burning
- damaging DNA
- destroying collagen
- causing premature skin ageing and wrinkles
- causing skin cancers

Who's most at risk? In general, the paler your skin, the more careful you have to be in the sun. The trouble is that a deep tan takes time to appear; some people can never manage it however often they sunbathe. Red-haired, freckly skinned people are the most vulnerable because they don't tan easily, if at all. Children, with their tender, delicate skin, are also especially at risk.

The deep tan that so many pale people crave is actually their skin's cry for help – a desperate attempt to protect itself against the UV rays. And don't make the mistake of thinking that if you have developed a nice tan you're safe against sun damage. Far from it. The deepest tan is no more effective than the flimsiest of sunscreens

(SPF2 to 4). Even black people get sunburned if they're not careful. The blackest skin has an SPF of 12 to 13, which is some way below the recommended minimum SPF for sunscreens of 15.

When and where is the sun most dangerous? The short answer is whenever and wherever there's less atmosphere between it and you to filter out the harmful UV rays.

Season, time of day and latitude are the key factors. In temperate zones like the UK the sun is most dangerous during the summer months when the sun is highest in the sky, particularly in the few hours around noon. Cornwall, with its miles of beaches and southern position, has the highest rates of skin cancer in the country. In tropical and subtropical zones, the danger is all year round and at most times of day. Pale-skinned people living, working or holidaying in these climes are most likely to be overexposed. Australia, for example, has one of the highest rates of skin cancer in the world – 50 per cent of the population has some form of it.

Another factor is altitude. The higher you are, the thinner the air and the less protection from the sun.

And the final factor is reflection. Sea, snow, shiny or white surfaces can reflect the sunlight and add to the UV rays, hence the need for special care when skiing, sailing, surfing or ironing sheets in the back garden on a sunny Monday morning.

Incidentally, light cloud offers very little protection, but heavy cloud and glass are quite good at filtering out the damaging rays.

Sunbeds and tanning studios

Every high street has its clutch of tanning studios or sunbed salons. They are seen as a quick and convenient way of getting or keeping a tan. But, like real sunlight, they use powerful UV rays which can cause premature ageing, skin cancer and eye damage if not used extremely carefully. They are currently unregulated and there are concerns that some salons don't adhere to approved guidelines and use staff who are not adequately trained.

Six steps to sun protection

Here are a few simple guidelines for when the sun is strong:

1 **Stay in the shade** Unless you are intent on getting a tan, spend more time in the shade, especially in a hot climate.

2 **Pick your moment** Avoid the hours around noon when the sun is highest and strongest.

3 **Cover up** Wear a wide-brimmed hat, long-sleeved shirt or top, long skirt or trousers, and wrap-around sunglasses. Admittedly not the quickest way to get a tan, but oh so sensible. Why wrap-around sunglasses? Because in really bright conditions a lot of UV rays can reach your eyes from around the sides of ordinary specs. (If, like me, you hate wrap-around sunglasses, forget it, but they're especially good for skiing.)

4 **Ration yourself** For serious sunbathing in hot sun, starting from scratch, allow yourself no more than about 15 to 20 minutes on each side, stopping at the first sign of pinkness. Your tan will be triggered by the first exposure and will develop over the next 3 days, even if the weather turns and you're stuck indoors playing dominoes. For a deeper tan, you'll need to spend more time in the sun.

5 **Use a sunscreen** You should use a broad-spectrum, water-resistant sunscreen with protection of at least SPF15 or, if your skin's really sensitive, a sunblock with titanium dioxide. Apply generously and frequently, especially after swimming and drying yourself with a towel. But don't make the mistake of thinking that, because you've got the sunscreen on, you can stay in the sun for much longer. The best way to tan is to expose yourself to the sun little and often.

6 **Check your skin** This is something for bathtime all the year round. Keep an eye out for sores that don't heal, pimples that look nasty and moles that start itching or growing. Check your partner too. If there's anything you're dubious about, show it to your GP without delay. See page 149.

Proper wrap-around eye protection and strict time limits are crucial, and people who have lots of freckles or moles or a history of skin cancer should avoid these facilities.

Heatstroke

Just a little too long on that Mediterranean beach – despite the lashings of sunscreen. An hour or two of being jostled in the crowds of a sweltering street market. A couple of beers with a leisurely lunch. Playing a few too many games of tennis or volleyball in the high heat of noon.

Heatstroke (sometimes called sunstroke) has a nasty habit of creeping up on people. The only warning may be a slight feeling of being 'out-of-sorts' with weariness and a headache, and then, quite suddenly, your temperature starts to shoot through the roof. This is a medical emergency needing urgent treatment. Heatstroke can kill.

You can prevent this disaster by staying cool and well hydrated. Wear light, loose clothing made of a natural material such as cotton that lets your perspiration evaporate. Spend more time in the shade, use a fan if you have one and avoid heavy exertion in the heat of the day. Drink plenty of bottled water or soft drinks and put extra salt on your food. And you could always consider having your holiday in Britain next year!

 The Sun Smart campaign, run by Cancer Research UK, has an excellent website at www.sunsmart.org.uk or telephone 020 7121 6699.

Things to think about when you get home

Always a welcome relief, however wonderful your trip. But there are still a few things to bear in mind.

Jet lag This is a problem with long flights in an east/west or west/east direction. You can minimise its effects by adopting home mealtimes and sleep–wake times as soon as you get back or, if you can, on the flight home.

Malaria If you were taking malaria tablets while abroad, keep doing so for a further month after returning.

Illness If you become ill, particularly with a fever or diarrhoea, tell your doctor which countries you've visited recently.

Risks If you were bitten by an animal, or risked catching a sexually transmitted infection, see your doctor for a check-up, even if you're feeling absolutely fine.

 For further information on health issues while travelling, visit the National Travel Health Network and Centre website at www.nathnac.org. The Department of Health – Health Advice for Travellers also provides information and advice at www.dhgov.uk.

Small changes, big difference

So far in this book we've been through some of the most important ways to boost your health and protect yourself against the slings and arrows of outrageous living.

But, however careful and sensible we are, things can, and perhaps all too often do, go wrong. A bit of wear-and-tear here. Slightly scratched paintwork there. Wobbly wheels. Bent axle. Worn bearings. Strange knocking noise. Uh oh.

So let's get mechanical. Let's talk about the sort of maintenance and check-ups we might need to head off some of the mid-life malfunctions that threaten to clobber our working parts.

Bodycheck

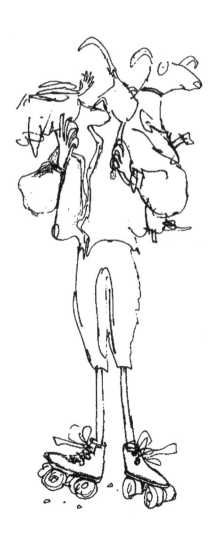

Considering how important our bodies are, most people are very lackadaisical about basic maintenance and check-ups. Too many of us are sloppy about oral health, ignore smear test invitations, don't bother to get our eyes tested or fail to turn up for breast screening. Men, in particular, are notoriously casual about this sort of thing (prevention, I mean). We look after our cars and front hedges better than our bodies.

Now that we're getting to an age when things start to go wrong or fall off, it's even more important to cherish what we still have and use every opportunity to spot problems as early as possible so that we can take action. Of course, we can take this idea too far and become a nation of hypochondriacs worried sick about our health. But if we just stick to the basics, we won't go far wrong.

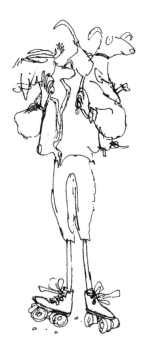

This chapter provides a simple maintenance and check-up schedule for the over-fifties. Here's a quick reference guide to direct you to the body-part you're most concerned with at the moment!

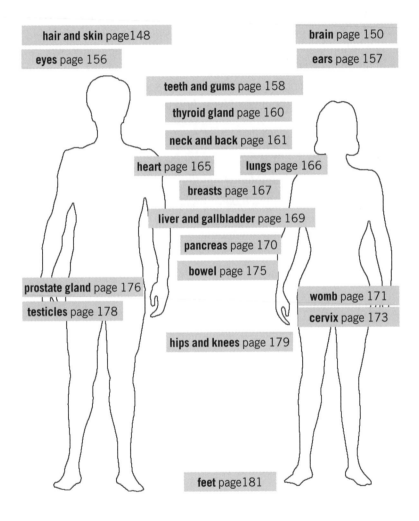

hair and skin page148

eyes page 156

brain page 150

ears page 157

teeth and gums page 158

thyroid gland page 160

neck and back page 161

heart page 165

lungs page 166

breasts page 167

liver and gallbladder page 169

pancreas page 170

bowel page 175

prostate gland page 176

testicles page 178

womb page 171

cervix page 173

hips and knees page 179

feet page181

Hair and skin

Well, what can I say? Zillions of words in magazines and newspapers are devoted to the subject of keeping our skin clear and youthful and our hair in tip-top condition. The whole beauty industry is geared to pamper and preen, buff and burnish, detox and exfoliate anything that moves. No matter that so many skin and hair products and services come wrapped in misleading pseudoscientific mumbo-jumbo. When all's said and done, they make us feel good about ourselves. And that's what really matters isn't it?

Well, yes and no. I think that too many people are being taken for a ride. It's upsetting to see so much hard-earned cash being wasted on expensive 'rejuvenating' skin care products that, frankly, are no more effective than a basic moisturiser, and on designer hair-care products that do no more than the high street, own-label versions.

Maintenance

From a simple good health point of view, routine skin and hair maintenance comes down to very little really – just pick and mix from water, soap, cleansing lotion, moisturiser, deodorant, mild shampoo and conditioner. That's more or less it. Perhaps you might need lip-salve and hand-cream. If you have a tendency to allergies or fungal infections, things become a little more complicated and you might need protective gloves for gardening and household chores.

Apart from routine cleanliness, the most important skin maintenance rules are to:

- eat a healthy balanced diet with plenty of fresh fruit and vegetables
- stop smoking
- take care in the sun
- protect your hands against detergents and other irritants

Check-ups

Middle age is the time when all sorts of odd changes start to happen to our skin. We develop wrinkles, age spots, pimples, thread veins and hairy moles, and our skin generally loses its elasticity. Hair too often changes, turning grey, becoming thinner, maybe with patchy loss.

If you're worried about any lumps, bumps or other changes, make an appointment to see your GP or practice nurse in the first instance. See your doctor immediately if you've found a mole that has changed in any of the 'ABCD' ways listed in the box below or if you've noticed:

- a new growth or sore that won't heal
- a spot, mole or sore that itches or hurts
- a mole or growth that bleeds, crusts or scabs

Mole watch – the ABCD check

See your GP or practice nurse straightaway if one of your moles shows any of the following signs:

A for Asymmetry: the two halves of your mole do not look the same.

B for Border: the edges of your mole are irregular, blurred or jagged.

C for Colour: the colour of your mole is uneven, with more than one shade.

D for Diameter: your mole is wider than 6mm in diameter (the width of a pencil).

The skin care campaign is an umbrella group for a number of organisations that provide information for the public and others about skin diseases and their treatment, and works to improve health care for people with skin diseases. The website lists helplines of member organisations (www.skincarecampaign.org).

Brain

Older and wiser – that's what I keep telling myself. And I'm beginning to think there might be some truth in it. The older bit is certainly right.

Speed of thinking

While our maturity and experience should, in theory at least, bring a degree of wisdom (been there, done that, got the mini-skirt or velvet flares to prove it), we can't always claim to have the quickness of brain or raw intelligence we possessed in our youth. Objective IQ tests, done against the clock, usually reveal a marked falling off in performance in people in their fifties and sixties. And although many older people are as sharp as a needle when it comes to thinking on their feet, more of us are beginning to lose that edge and their cogs are turning much more slowly. This can create problems when trying to do several things at once. Multi-tasking can be a bit too much for some people.

Senior moments

Another familiar problem is the 'senior moment', when you just can't quite remember someone's name, even though you know them so well. And then, a few minutes later, when the conversation has moved on, suddenly you've got it. This is not only inconvenient and perhaps embarrassing, it might also be important, particularly if it's your neighbour, boss or better half.

Memory does deteriorate to some extent in later life, but it tends to be the short-term memory that goes – what you did yesterday, this morning or, most worryingly, a few moments ago. The famous 'oh dear, did I turn off the gas?' syndrome. Memories from way back, especially childhood, are usually firmly lodged and easily retrievable.

People in middle age who are becoming a bit forgetful often worry that it could be the beginnings of Alzheimer's disease. But this is most unlikely. Alzheimer's is predominantly a disease of people who are over 75. Although cases do occur in the sixties, fifties and even forties, these are comparatively rare. Our senior moments are nearly always precisely that – lapses of memory caused by the steady loss of grey matter that tends to go with increasing age and is hastened in some cases by years of heavy drinking and drug use.

Speed and distance

What about our ability to judge speed and distance, and our general spatial awareness, particularly when it comes to driving? Do these go down the pan too? Well, I'm afraid to say that, as with IQ and memory, objective testing shows that these skills do tend to deteriorate in middle life and worsen as we get older.

Zest for life

Finally, what of our mood, our spirits, our zest for life? Surely we can at least feel good about ourselves? Yes, indeed we can – and that's the subject of the next chapter. But an awful lot of people in middle age suffer from depression in one form or another (see page 154) and this is a particularly common problem in women going through the menopause (see page 171).

Maintenance

Is there anything we can do to fend off this seemingly inexorable decline? Can we sharpen our thinking, improve our memory and develop our spatial skills?

Yes, yes, yes. Even though our brain is losing thousands of irreplaceable neurones every day (and has been doing so since our twenties), there are ways of compensating for this loss by making the best of what we've still got.

Sharpening thinking

There are hundreds of ways of sharpening our thinking, not least through spending time in the company of bright young things. Most of us have to be pretty sharp to keep up with the rapid-fire banter of our children or grandchildren. But doing quizzes, puzzles, crosswords or sudoku against the clock are also good brain-sharpening pastimes, as are card games requiring high levels of concentration and quick reactions.

Anything that requires you to think quickly and clearly will help to exercise your mind. It's not so much about knowledge, as about speed of thought and decision-making.

Improving memory

Do you have trouble remembering phone numbers or often find yourself struggling to put a name to a face? Me too.

Numbers Mobile phones with their contacts directory have helped hugely with the numbers problem. I assiduously add more and more numbers to mine, and dread to think what would happen to my life if I lost it. But some numbers cry out to be committed to memory – your own, for instance – and it's worth using a few simple techniques for making this easier:

Chunking – split the number into bite-sized chunks.

Patterns – see if there are any internal repeats, series, rhymes, sums or famous dates in the number.

Imaging – convert chunks of the number into images using a rhyming code such as: 1 (bun), 2 (shoe), 3 (tree), 4 (door), 5 (hive), six (sticks), 7 (heaven), 8 (gate), 9 (twine), 0 (hero). For 743, you could picture heaven with a door and a tree, which is easy as long as you get the order right. It would be no good picturing a tree with a door in heaven. (Hmmm, not so sure about this method. I'll need to practise.)

Names and faces Names and faces are more difficult. Repeating someone's name as soon as you've been introduced to them is a help. So too is silently testing yourself for half an hour afterwards. You could also try a form of imaging in which you think of a good friend with the same forename and imagine them dancing together. It's amazing how well this can work. Or try using rhyming words and imagery together – for example, Lucinda could be 'cinders' and you picture her as Cinderella with a broomstick or you imagine Robin with a redbreasted bird on his shoulder.

Other memory aids Other tried and tested aids include:

- Lists (I have so many lists, I have to keep a list of my lists).
- Cues to remind you to do something important (tying a knot in your hankie, putting your watch on the other wrist or standing your radio on the front doormat).
- Routines where you always do the same things in the same way in the same methodical order, day in, day out, year in, year out. Men tend to like this one. It drives my dear wife bonkers.

Developing spatial skills

This is all about judging distance, speed and space – hand-eye co-ordination. There are countless ways to keep up your skills. Driving is one. Dancing is another, and so is any ball game. Indeed, most sports require spatial skills. All the more reason to keep active, particularly with something as spatial as, say, tennis or golf. For me, it's weaving my way through city traffic on my pushbike.

Check-ups

The most common mental assessment undertaken by GPs is a brief checklist for symptoms and signs of depression. This is, in effect, a set of questions that help to reveal whether someone might need antidepressant medication or a 'talking treatment' such as counselling or cognitive behavioural therapy (CBT) from a psychotherapist, psychologist or psychiatrist.

Another assessment is for Alzheimer's disease and the other forms of dementia. Again, this comes in the form of a questionnaire which looks for signs of loss of cognitive ability (thinking, reasoning and memory).

Both of these assessments should be accompanied by a full physical examination to check for possible causes such as the menopause, depression, an underactive thyroid, diabetes, stroke or, more often than not, the side-effects of medication.

For further information MIND is the leading independent mental health organisation with over 200 local groups across England and Wales. The MIND infoline offers confidential help on a range of mental health issues (telephone 0845 766 0163; www.mind.org.uk).

SAMH is the leading mental health charity in Scotland (telephone 0141 568 7000; www.samh.org.uk).

NIAMH provides local support for people with mental health needs across Northern Ireland (telephone 028 9032 8474; www.niamh.co.uk).

Depression

We all get a bit down from time to time. Money worries, relationship problems, disappointments, trouble at work, or the bitter blow of losing a loved one. But these normal feelings of sadness, perhaps a very deep and lasting sadness, don't necessarily amount to clinical depression. We feel very low, but we carry on.

What doctors call depression, or rather depressive illness, is when the drive to carry on is lost. As well as the low mood, many other aspects of normal function may be affected, so that carrying on in any proper functioning way becomes very difficult. To someone with depression, everything feels dreadful – like being weighed down by a huge heavy blanket made of black lead. There is no joy whatsoever. No purpose. No reason to get up. No light at the end of the tunnel. It is utter misery and many sufferers feel there's no real reason to carry on at all. They look to suicide as a way out.

Symptoms might include any or all of the following:

- sleep disturbance
- agitation
- loss of confidence
- tearfulness
- lack of appetite
- loss of sex drive
- difficulty concentrating
- slowness of thought
- loss of memory
- self-harm and suicidal thoughts

Many things can trigger depressive illness. It can follow any of the normal crises mentioned above. It also commonly accompanies the menopause, an underactive thyroid, alcohol dependence, stroke and ageing.

One of the commonest triggers is the 'empty nest syndrome', when the children finally leave home. Another is SAD (seasonal affective disorder), caused by a reaction to lack of sunlight during the winter. Depression can also occur for no apparent reason – some inexplicable change in the brain's chemistry that seems to appear out of the blue.

Whatever the trigger, the important thing is to recognise it early, before any harm can be done, and for the person to use a combination of talking treatment and medication to help themselves get back to full health.

 Contact the Samaritans for confidential emotional support, 24 hours a day, 7 days a week (telephone 08457 90 90 90; www.samaritans.org).

Eyes

One of the signs of middle age is the need for reading glasses. It happens because the lenses in our eyes become stiffer and are less able to focus on near things. Reading small print, threading a needle and wiring a plug become difficult without a bright light and very long arms.

Another change for some people is dry eyes. Their tear-glands produce less tear-fluid and their eyes feel tired and gritty.

A third common problem, especially a bit later on in life, is cataracts – gradual patchy clouding of the lenses causing dullness of vision. Cataracts are mainly due to natural ageing, but are sometimes caused by overexposure to strong sunlight over a period of years.

Changes may also happen to the internal pressure of the eyeballs (glaucoma), or to the retina (screen at the back of the eye) owing to high blood pressure or diabetes.

Maintenance

What should we be doing to keep our eyes shiny and bright? Surprisingly, not a lot. Our eyes do most of the regular maintenance work for us. We can help by bathing our eyelids with warm water, removing make-up at night, avoiding strong sunlight and glare, staying away from smoky atmospheres, and taking care with contact lenses. But all those eyecare solutions really are just eyewash.

Check-ups

The advice is to visit your optician to have your eyes tested at least once every 2 years, or more often if necessary. Take along any specs or contacts and a note of your medications. As well as checking your vision, the optometrist will also look at your natural lenses for signs of cataract, your irises to make sure they react properly to light and your retinas to look for abnormalities. You should also have the pressure in your eyeballs checked – usually done with a rather clever machine that puffs a little pulse of air at them. Completely non-invasive and painless. Don't ask me how it works.

You're entitled to free NHS eye tests if:

- you're aged 60 or over
- you or your partner receive various benefits (check with your optician)
- you have diabetes or glaucoma (or are at risk of glaucoma)
- you're 40 or over and have a close relative with glaucoma
- you're registered blind or partially sighted
- you're entitled to vouchers for complex lenses

These rules change from time to time, so it's best to check with your optician before you have the eye test.

 For further information on eye-related issues, contact the Eyecare Trust, which is run by the ophthalmic professions (telephone 0845 129 5001; www.eye-care.org.uk). The RNIB is the UK's leading charity offering information, support and advice to over 2 million people with sight problems (telephone helpline 0845 766 9999; www.rnib.org.uk).

Ears

As we get older, our ears are more likely to become clogged with hard wax. If this happens, ask the pharmacist for some eardrops to soften it. Persistent wax may need syringing by your practice nurse.

Other common problems in middle age include tinnitus (abnormal ringing or buzzing in one or both ears) and difficulty hearing, particularly higher notes and speech.

Maintenance

Like eyes, ears are pretty good at looking after themselves as long as we don't abuse them. Apart from soap and water, they're best left to their own devices. Indeed, our ears have a particularly brilliant way of getting rid of all the dust and grime that accumulates during the day. The lining of the ear canal traps the detritus in its soft wax coating, which continually and very gradually edges its way out of the ear, carrying all the gunge with it. An occasional wipe with a tissue is usually all that's needed. Never be tempted to probe into the ear canal with an orange stick or cotton bud. You'll risk introducing infection or rupturing the delicate eardrum.

Check-ups

Routine testing usually isn't necessary. But if you think you might have partial loss of hearing or are worried about your ears for any other reason, it's best to visit your GP in the first instance.

The RNID is a national charity that aims to make daily life better for deaf and hard of hearing people through campaigns, information, services and supporting research (information freephone 0808 808 0123; www.rnid.org.uk).

Teeth and gums

Thirty years ago, four out of ten adults in the UK had no natural teeth. Today it's less than half that figure, thanks largely to better oral hygiene and dental check-ups. But it's still the case that too many older people are losing their teeth unnecessarily.

The main problem in later life is inflammation of the gums, which can soon develop into full-blown gum disease. Also known as gingivitis, gum disease is caused by plaque, the sticky yellow coating of bacteria, collecting in the nooks and crannies of the mouth, especially between the teeth. Tartar or calculus (the limescale deposit) may also play a part. The first sign of a problem is slight bleeding when you brush.

Soon, pockets develop between the gum and the teeth. These pockets are difficult to keep clean and act as a haven for bacteria-laden plaque and calculus. Over a period of years the inflammation slowly spreads deeper. Eventually, the gum recedes and the tooth anchorages become loosened. It doesn't take much to push the tooth out.

Another problem is tooth decay at the gum margins, where the gums have receded and the soft yellow dentine is exposed. This is vulnerable to attack by acid plaque.

And a third common problem is halitosis – bad breath. Again this is mostly caused by plaque in the gum pockets, but it's sometimes aggravated by a lack of saliva.

Maintenance

- Give special attention to good oral hygiene – brushing, flossing and mouthwashing.
- Brush twice daily with a small-headed, medium toothbrush, using small strokes at an angle to the gum margin to reach the tufts into any pockets. An electric toothbrush may make this easier.
- Use dental floss or tape once daily to clean between the teeth. If you find this too fiddly, try an interdental brush or special wooden stick.
- Brush your tongue to help reduce halitosis.
- Rinse with antiseptic mouthwash.
- Avoid eating and drinking sugary things – these provide fodder for plaque.

Check-ups

Make sure you have an oral check-up and descale at least once every 6 months.

For free dental advice, contact the British Dental Health Foundation, an independent charity working to bring about improved standards of oral healthcare (telephone helpline 0845 063 1188 (Monday to Friday, 9am to 5pm); www.dentalhealth.org.uk).

Thyroid gland

This gland, situated around the base of the Adam's Apple, produces important hormones. Problems with the thyroid often develop in middle age, especially in women. The most common are hypothyroidism (underactive thyroid) or hyperthyroidism (overactive thyroid). Either way, you feel awful.

With an underactive thyroid you become very tired, slow in thought and action, forgetful, overweight, puffy faced, coarse-haired and gruff-voiced, although most people don't have all these symptoms and some may only have one or two of them slightly.

With an overactive thyroid, you become tense, jumpy, nervy and tearful. You lose your appetite and turn into a thin shaky wraith with a fluttering heart. Again, you might not have all of these symptoms – perhaps just one or two of them slightly.

Maintenance

These problems arise out of the blue, usually as a so-called auto-immune disorder in which the immune system attacks the body's own cells. This is a relatively common occurrence in middle-aged women, often linked to the menopause.

Check-ups

Your doctor will take a sample of blood to measure the levels of the key hormones.

If you are concerned about a thyroid disorder, the British Thyroid Foundation provides a range of information and support (telephone 01423 709 707; www.btf-thyroid.org).

Neck and back

When you consider how many bits there are to go wrong in the average person's spine, it's amazing that it manages to prop us up so well. There are 26 separate bones: 7 cervical (neck) vertebrae; 12 thoracic (chest) vertebrae; 5 lumbar vertebrae; the sacrum (back of the pelvis); and the coccyx (tailbone). We've got nearly as many spinal discs acting as shock absorbers between the vertebrae, dozens of ligaments strapping the skull, ribs and pelvis to the vertebrae and the vertebrae to each other, and dozens more muscles and tendons acting as guy-ropes, winches and cranes. It's an amazingly complex structure and a miracle of engineering. And the remarkable fact is that it has evolved over hundreds of thousands of years just so that we can stand up on our hind legs and hit a small white ball into a hole.

But unfortunately there's a price to be paid for this evolution. Nearly everyone suffers from neck pain or backache at some time in their lives. And it happens more often as we get older. Here are some tips on how to avoid most of the trouble that comes with being an upright citizen.

Maintenance – neck

Most of the problems in the neck are due to muscle strain. Your head is a surprisingly heavy item, balanced on top of a very slender column of bones and held in place by sensitive ligaments and muscles. The latter spend most of the day clenched hard, trying to keep your head in position and pointing in the right direction. No wonder that they ache after a while and develop tender knots and nodules – trigger points of pain. Sedentary workers are particularly vulnerable to these types of problems, sitting all day with their head tipped forward and their neck and shoulder muscles rigid with tension. Sometimes the pain and spasm extend over the scalp and into the forehead.

To help avoid these problems, make sure your seat, desk or work surface is properly adjusted so that your head doesn't have to lean forward. Second, if you can, rest your head on your hand to provide extra support. Third, take frequent breaks, stretch, stand up, walk around, roll your shoulders, rotate your neck and generally loosen up.

Another common problem is caused by wear and tear on the discs in the neck (cervical spondylosis). This causes pressure on the nerve roots, giving rise to shooting pains, pins and needles and muscle spasm in the neck, back of the head, shoulders or arms. Most people over 50 have a certain degree of cervical spondylosis, and you're most likely to become aware of it if you carry heavy shopping or lug heavy flowerpots or bags of compost around the garden. It might also become apparent if your head is unsupported during sex.

You can avoid aggravating a troublesome neck by being careful about how you carry stuff, making sure that it's in small loads and evenly balanced in both hands or, better still, placed in a backpack or trolley. This approach is obviously less helpful during sex – try resting your head on a pillow and adopting a more passive mode.

Maintenance – back

By far the most common cause of backache is a pulled muscle or strained ligament in the lumbar region (small of the back). When you think how heavy the upper half of your body is, you can imagine how extreme the forces on your lower spine must be, especially when you bend to lift a heavy object. If these forces are too great, or too sudden, you'll either pull something in your back or 'slip' a disc. I put the word 'slip' in inverted commas because the disc doesn't really slip. It bursts.

The discs between the vertebrae act like heavy-duty cushions. Their job is to stop the vertebrae grinding and crunching on each other and to absorb any shocks, impacts, twists and bends. Each disc comprises a tough, leathery, disc-shaped bag with a soft gel-filled centre. Whenever you sit, stand, bend or lift something, the pressure on the soft centres of the lumbar discs can be immense. If the pressure is too great, the leathery ring bursts and the soft gel is squeezed out, like toothpaste, into the spinal canal. This is extremely painful, causing acute back pain and muscle spasm. If the extruded gel presses on nerve roots, the result is likely to be sciatica, a dreadful sharp pain in the buttock and down the back of the leg.

People most at risk of a slipped disc are those who spend all day sitting down and then suddenly do some heavy lifting and shifting. The office worker who decides to lay some crazy paving at the weekend. The person loading heavy shopping into the hatchback or helping their daughter move furniture into a new flat. But if your discs are getting a bit frayed, as they usually are in later life, the slightest thing can do it – an awkward stumble, a sudden twist, even a violent sneeze.

How can a slipped disc be avoided? By being very careful how you bend and lift heavy or awkward things, and paying special attention to how you sit.

Lifting and carrying

If you have to lift a heavy object from the ground, don't bend forwards at the waist. Crouch down, keeping your back straight; then, holding the load as closely as possible, straighten up again.

If you have to turn to one side holding something heavy, don't twist at the waist. Instead, turn your feet.

If you have to carry something heavy or awkward, try to get someone to help you or use a wheelbarrow or trolley. You might be able to drag the object or 'walk' it without having to lift it.

Make sure any load is stable. If it suddenly slips and you lurch, you'll be risking a pulled muscle or slipped disc.

Don't lean too far into a car boot with a heavy load. Get it onto the ledge and slide it forward. Reverse this procedure when unloading.

Bending, sitting, lying

Bending forwards for a long time – weeding the garden, for example – puts a huge strain on your back muscles. Better to get down on one or both knees, using a kneeling mat, spare bit of carpet or even a pile of folded newspapers.

If you spend a lot of time sitting, make sure your chair is at the right height. If you're at a desk, a swivel office chair with an adjustable backrest is best. Sit upright and don't slouch.

When sitting in an easy chair, make sure your lower back is well supported with cushions.

At night, a firm mattress is usually best for a bad back. If you've got an old saggy mattress, get rid of it and invest in something more supportive, with pocketed springs if you can afford them. Here's a simple test to check the suitability of your mattress. Lie on your back and slide your hand (palm down) under the small of your back. If there's a large gap, the mattress is probably too hard. If you have to force your hand under your back, it's probably too soft. If your hand slides in fairly easily, the mattress is probably about right.

Exercising

One of the best forms of aerobic exercise if you have a dodgy back is swimming. You can do lengths and build up your fitness without jolting or straining your back. For more static exercises, try pilates (see page 42). Just right for bad backs.

For further information about how to prevent and manage neck and back pain, contact BackCare, an independent national charity that provides information, publications and a helpline. It also promotes best practice, funds research and runs local self-help branches through the country (telephone helpline 0845 130 2704; www.backpain.org).

Heart

By far the main threat to the middle-aged heart is coronary disease – clogging of the coronary arteries, the narrow arteries (no wider than a drinking straw) that branch over the surface of the heart and supply the heart muscle itself. Over a period of many years these tend to silt up with a cholesterol-rich fatty deposit, and this can all too often lead to angina pain and a heart attack.

Maintenance

This is all about keeping active, eating healthily, relaxing and stopping smoking. We covered all these pretty thoroughly earlier, so let's focus here on basic heart-health check-ups, sometimes called cardiovascular risk assessments.

Check-ups

Apart from checking your weight, which we talked about in 'Watching your weight', here are the three basic checks that your GP is likely to do if you haven't been along for a while.

Blood pressure

There are two measurements. The upper figure is your systolic pressure (peak of the pulse wave), and the lower figure is your diastolic pressure (trough of the pulse wave). The higher your blood pressure, the greater the risk of stroke, heart disease and kidney disease. The usual definition of hypertension is blood pressure persistently at or above 140/90. You can help to keep your blood pressure down by eating less salt, watching your weight, keeping active, cutting down on alcohol and coping with stress.

Blood cholesterol (or lipids)

This is a blood test, either by fingerprick or, for a more accurate reading, a sample from a vein. As well as total cholesterol, the test usually measures LDL cholesterol ('bad' cholesterol), HDL cholesterol ('good' cholesterol), and triglycerides (another fatty substance in your blood). You can help to keep your LDL cholesterol under control by cutting down on fatty foods, especially saturated fats, and being more active.

Blood sugar (glucose)

This is a blood test, from fingerprick or vein, usually taken after fasting for 12 hours. The result should be between 4 and 6 units. Higher than 7 suggests diabetes.

 For information about heart disease, contact the British Heart Foundation (telephone 08450 70 80 70; www.bhf.org.uk).

Lungs

Lungs are our vital bellows, silently working away without our having to spare them a thought – until they go wrong. Problems include:

* Asthma, which can occur for the first time in middle age. Often triggered by smoking.

* Chronic bronchitis. Chronic bronchitis together with emphysema is now called COPD – chronic obstructive pulmonary disease. Big improvement I'm sure you'll agree. Usually caused by smoking.

* Lung cancer. Nearly always caused by smoking.

Maintenance

I'm just going to say one thing, and you know what it is. If you're a smoker, give your lungs a chance to survive another few years. Stop filling them with tar, soot, carbon monoxide, cyanide, polyphenols and dozens of other toxins and pollutants. Help with giving up smoking begins on page 119.

Check-ups

Two tests commonly used by GPs to check your lungs are:

Peak-flow meter This is a simple device for measuring how clear and open your airways are. You simply breathe out through your mouth as fast as you can. The peak-flow meter is useful for monitoring asthma.

Carbon monoxide monitor This is another simple breathing-out device. This one measures the carbon monoxide in your system – a quick check of your recent smoking level.

 For information about lung disease, contact the British Lung Foundation (telephone helpline 08458 50 50 20; www.lunguk.org).

Breasts

Every woman fears breast cancer, especially in her older years when it becomes much more common.

Maintenance

This is really just about being aware of how your breasts normally look and feel at different times, so that you can recognise any changes that are unusual for you and report them to your doctor without delay.

The Department of Health does not recommend routine self-examination as a set technique because there's no scientific evidence to show that regular methodical self-examination is any more effective than general awareness. What is important, if you're over 50, is to make sure you have your mammogram every 3 years.

Check-ups

The purpose of breast screening is to detect an actual cancer as early as possible so that treatment can be most effective. The initial check-up involves a low-dose x-ray of each breast – a mammogram – taken while carefully compressing the breast between two plastic plates. Most women find this a bit uncomfortable and a few find it painful, but it's an important check-up to have because the mammogram can detect clues of a possible cancer long before it's big enough for either you or your doctor to feel it.

The latest technique takes two x-rays of each breast – one from above and one diagonally across the breast towards the armpit. Research has shown that this additional 'view' makes the mammogram much better at detecting really small cancers.

The NHS breast screening programme provides free breast screening every 3 years for all women in the UK aged 50 and over. Women aged between 50 and 70 are now routinely invited. However, because it's a rolling programme which invites groups of women area by area, you might not receive your invitation until you're 51 or 52. As with the cervical screening programme, invitations are based on GP lists. It's therefore crucial that you are registered with a GP and the practice has your correct contact details.

When you're over 70, the automatic invitations will cease, but you are encouraged to make your own 3-yearly appointments, still free on the NHS. I would strongly advise you to keep up the regular screening because the risk of breast cancer continues to increase as you get older.

Since the national programme began in 1988, it has successfully detected well over 100,000 cases of cancer. Every year around 1.5 million women are screened in the UK, saving over 1,500 lives.

Further information about the NHS breast screening programme can be found at www.cancerscreening.nhs.uk/breastscreen. Breast screening is also offered by a number of private and independent healthcare providers.

Information and support for those affected by breast cancer are available from Breast Cancer Care (telephone helpline 0808 800 6000; www.breastcancercare.org.uk). NHS Direct (telephone 0845 4647; www.nhsdirect.nhs.uk) also provides a range of information.

Liver and gallbladder

The liver is the body's much abused chemical factory and natural built-in detox unit. It's the liver's job to dismantle and render harmless most of the wicked or worrying substances that find their way into our bloodstream via our digestive system, including, of course, alcohol. And it is indeed alcohol, friend and foe, that is the greatest threat to the nation's livers.

It's also the liver's job to make bile, the digestive juice stored in the gallbladder. Gallstones, which very commonly form in the bile in the gallbladder, especially in middle-aged women, can cause a blockage and give rise to severe pain and jaundice.

Maintenance

Be sensible. Drink sensibly. Read the sobering advice starting on page 123.

Check-ups

Your GP will feel your tummy for the tell-tale firm edge of an enlarged liver, and order a blood test to check the level of enzymes that reveal liver damage. Another blood test will give an early warning of a blocked bile duct. An x-ray or ultrasound will show gallstones.

Information and advice for people who are concerned about liver disease is available from the British Liver Trust (telephone 0870 770 8028; www.britishlivertrust.org.uk).

Pancreas

Your pancreas is a dual-function gland just beneath your stomach. One job is to make pancreatic enzymes which are squirted into the duodenum and help to digest your food. The other is to make insulin – the hormone that is so important in controlling the level of glucose in your bloodstream.

Diabetes

In some people the pancreas fails to make enough insulin, leading to a dangerous rise in blood glucose. This is type 1 diabetes, usually beginning in children and younger people. A much more common form of diabetes, type 2, affects mainly middle-aged and older people. It occurs when, for some reason, the body fails to respond properly to the insulin that is being made. The pancreas produces plenty of insulin but the blood glucose rises anyway. This is a frequent complication of obesity.

The main symptoms of uncontrolled type 2 diabetes are excessive tiredness, lack of energy, unusual thirst, passing more water than usual, unexplained weight loss, pins and needles, frequent attacks of thrush, boils or other infections, and, in extreme cases, coma. It's a potentially serious condition that can eventually cause circulatory problems, heart attacks, kidney disease and impaired vision.

Maintenance

Fortunately, type 2 diabetes can usually be well-controlled by eating a healthy balanced diet, watching your weight and, in some cases, taking glucose-lowering medication.

Check-ups

A simple dipstick test will check whether there is glucose in your urine. This could indicate a raised level of glucose in the blood. Urine should be completely sugar-free. If glucose is detected, you should have a blood test to measure the level in your bloodstream.

Blood tests are usually a self-administered fingerprick test, using a pen-like device that gives a rapid read-out, or carried out by a doctor or nurse taking a sample of blood in a syringe. Sometimes the blood test is done after the person has been fasting for at least 8 hours (fasting blood sugar).

A wide range of information on diabetes is available from Diabetes UK, which aims to improve the care, treatment and quality of life for people with diabetes. The charity's careline is staffed by trained counsellors (telephone 0845 120 2960 (Monday to Friday, 9am to 5pm); www.diabetes.org.uk).

Womb

A woman's early fifties are often dominated by the menopause – the 'change of life' when the hormones diminish, the ovaries cease to produce eggs, the periods stop, and the womb shrinks into a state of serene indifference. At least, that's what's meant to happen. The reality can be very different.

Four out of five women sail through the menopause with little or no bother at all. Their periods become less regular and lighter, although perhaps with occasional heavier 'floods'. Eventually, after an average of about 5 years of this winding down, they stop altogether.

But it's really the other symptoms of the menopause that can cause most problems – the hot flushes, night drenches, mood swings, panic attacks, agoraphobia, vaginal dryness, thrush, cystitis, irritable bowel, headaches, palpitations, lank hair, blemished skin and osteoporosis, to mention but a few.

Maintenance

Here are some tried and tested self-help tips to make your menopause a little easier.

Hot flushes Try to avoid triggers like very hot drinks, spicy foods and airless rooms. A fan can be a real comfort, especially in summer.

Vaginal dryness Use a lubricant jelly from the high street pharmacist. You can also buy antifungal cream or suppositories for thrush (if you're reasonably sure it is thrush) over the counter.

Mood swings Try to see this as a phase that will soon pass, even though it seems to be dragging on for ever. Remind yourself of all the positives in your life. Become more active. Make an effort to follow the advice in 'Stressing less'. It really will help. Your family and friends should understand what you're going through and give you the support you need.

Check-ups

Continuing heavy periods will need to be properly investigated, and your doctor will refer you to a gynaecologist for a womb scan and other check-ups. A common problem is fibroids, which might need surgical treatment, although they usually shrink to nothing during the menopause.

The big issue for many women is whether to have HRT (hormone replacement therapy). Because of the potential risks of thrombosis and other problems, this is now usually only prescribed when menopausal symptoms are severe and for a much shorter period of time than in the past. If you would like to consider HRT, ask your doctor to give you the pros and cons as they apply in your particular case. You will need to have a cardiovascular check-up before starting the therapy (see 'Heart' on page 165).

Information on the menopause is available from the Menopause Amarant Trust, which provides a range of services, including a nurse-staffed helpline (www. amarantmenopausetrust.org.uk).

Cervix

The cervix (neck of the womb) is commonly infected with HPV – the human papilloma virus that causes genital warts, a sexually transmitted infection. Some strains of the virus are linked to an increased risk of cervical cancer.

HPV infection is extremely common, but cervical cancer is relatively rare. About 80 per cent of women have been infected with HPV by the age of 50, but the great majority of these infections disappear without causing any problems. Even those women who contract a high-risk strain of HPV rarely go on to develop cervical cancer.

Check-ups

There are two ways of checking for the risk of cervical cancer – the smear test and the HPV test. Some experts say that women should have both check-ups.

The smear test

Also known as the 'pap test' or cervical screening, this is a way of detecting cell changes in the cervix, which, if left untreated, could eventually lead to cancer. The test involves having a sample of cells swept from the cervix and sent to the lab for examination under the microscope. The latest technique, using a very soft brush instead of a spatula, provides a better sample and has reduced the need for some women to have a repeat.

Recent changes to the programme mean that, if you're between the ages of 50 and 64, you'll now normally be invited to have the test every 5 years rather than every 3 years as has been the case. Women aged 65 and over are not invited for screening unless they haven't been screened since the age of 50 or have had recent abnormal test results.

The programme is highly effective and prevents 70 to 75 per cent of cervical cancers. However, because only women on GP lists are invited, it's absolutely crucial to make sure you're registered with a local practice and that they have your correct contact details.

The HPV test

This may prove to be a useful additional check-up for older women. HPV infection tends to be rarer but more persistent in older women, and it's important to know whether it's one of the high-risk strains.

Further information about the NHS cervical screening programme can be found at www.cancerscreening.nhs.uk/cervical. Cervical screening is also offered by a number of private and independent healthcare providers.

Information and support for those affected by cancer are available from a number of charities, including: Cancerbackup (telephone freephone 0808 800 1234 (Monday to Friday, 9am to 8pm); www.cancerbackup.org.uk); Cancer Research UK (www.cancerhelp.org.uk); Marie Curie Cancer Care (www.MarieCurie.org.uk); and Macmillan Cancer Support (telephone freephone 0808 808 2020 (Monday to Friday, 9am to 10pm); www.macmillan.org.uk). NHS Direct (telephone 0845 4647; www.nhsdirect.nhs.uk) also provides a range of information.

Bowel

As we get older we're more likely to experience bowel complaints such as constipation, piles and diverticular disease.

We're also more vulnerable to bowel cancer (also known as rectal, colon or colorectal cancer), the second most common type of cancer in both sexes. About one in 20 people in the UK will develop bowel cancer during their lifetime, mostly over the age of 50. It's the third most common cancer in the UK and the second leading cause of cancer death. Regular screening for bowel cancer, using the faecal occult blood test (FOB), significantly reduces this risk by detecting potential problems before symptoms appear, allowing treatment to be started much earlier, with a much better chance of cure.

Maintenance

For these reasons, it's particularly important for the over-fifties to eat plenty of high-fibre foods such as cereals, fruit and vegetables.

Check-ups

The NHS bowel cancer screening programme is currently being rolled out across the country. The programme offers a free screening test every 2 years to all men and women aged 60 to 69 in the areas where the test is available. People who wish to take part are sent an FOB test kit with step-by-step instructions on how to collect and return a sample of their stools. The test can detect traces of blood, invisible to the naked eye, which might be caused by various things, not just cancer. If the result is positive, further investigation is needed to confirm the diagnosis

As with the cervical and breast screening programmes, the invitations are based on GP lists, so it's important that you're registered with a GP and the practice has your correct contact details. People over 70 can request the kit for themselves.

Further information about the NHS bowel screening programme can be found at www.cancerscreening.nhs. uk/bowel. Bowel screening is also offered by a number of private and independent healthcare providers.

Information and support for those affected by cancer are available from a number of charities, including: Cancerbackup (telephone freephone 0808 800 1234 (Monday to Friday, 9am to 8pm); www.cancerbackup. org.uk); Cancer Research UK (www.cancerhelp.org. uk); Marie Curie Cancer Care (www.MarieCurie.org.uk); and Macmillan Cancer Support (telephone freephone 0808 808 2020 (Monday to Friday, 9am to 10pm); www.macmillan.org.uk). NHS Direct (telephone 0845 4647; www.nhsdirect.nhs.uk) also provides a range of information.

Prostate gland

This is a men-only gland, normally about the size and shape of a chestnut, located just beneath the bladder. The outlet pipe from the bladder passes right through it and is joined by tubes from the testicles carrying sperm. The gland's job is to make seminal fluid, the salty liquid that the sperm swims in during ejaculation.

The prostate gland very gradually enlarges in later life, which is a normal part of the ageing process. Problems arise if the swollen gland tissue constricts the urethra and bulges into the bladder, distorting its outlet valve. The symptoms, very mild to begin with, can become a major nuisance for middle-aged and older men, causing the need to pee several times during the night, difficulty getting started and dribbling incontinence.

Check-ups

The simplest check-up for an enlarged prostate is a rectal examination. Your doctor should be able to feel the enlarged gland very easily and organise the appropriate treatment.

More of a worry is prostate cancer, the third most common cancer in men after lung and bowel, and more likely to occur in the over-fifties (especially in the over-seventies). There is no very satisfactory screening test for prostate cancer. The nearest thing is the PSA (prostate-specific antigen) blood test. But this is only a general pointer and a long way from being a clear-cut test. Sometimes a raised PSA level can be a sign of prostate cancer, although it's more likely to be caused by something less serious like an inflamed or enlarged prostate. It's also worth remembering that, in most cases, prostate cancer is very slow growing, particularly in older men, and the treatment can be more troublesome than the disease. The best advice is to check out the information sources below and talk the pros and cons over with your GP.

Information and support for people concerned about prostate problems are available from the Prostate Research Campaign UK (telephone 020 8877 5840; www.prostate-research.org.uk). Information about the NHS prostate cancer risk management programme can be found at www.cancerscreening.nhs.uk/prostate.

Information and support for those affected by cancer are available from a number of charities, including: Cancerbackup (telephone freephone 0808 800 1234 (Monday to Friday, 9am to 8pm); www.cancerbackup. org.uk); Cancer Research UK (www.cancerhelp.org. uk); Marie Curie Cancer Care (www.MarieCurie.org.uk); and Macmillan Cancer Support (telephone freephone 0808 808 2020 (Monday to Friday, 9am to 10pm); www.macmillan.org.uk). NHS Direct (telephone 0845 4647; www.nhsdirect.nhs.uk) also provides a range of information.

Testicles

When you think about how delicate and vulnerable they are, it's amazing that most men manage to get to middle age without some major mishap. But apart from trauma, there are few things that can go wrong with the testicles. Some men have difficulty producing normal sperm, which causes infertility. But abnormal lumps are the main concern, most of which (such as a varicocele – a knot of swollen veins) are non-cancerous.

Maintenance

Little or no maintenance is required. The testicles' shyness and slipperiness seems to keep them out of most trouble. Men who have been told they have subfertile sperm should avoid hot baths and tight jeans.

Check-ups

The testicles are so easily palpable, there's really no excuse for men not to check them from time to time. It's best done in or after a shower or bath when the scrotum is loose. Feel carefully round each testicle, which should be smooth, except at the top and back where it will normally be rather uneven where the coiled sperm tube enters. Various disorders can cause lumps in the scrotum, including cancer. Testicular cancers are more common in younger men. About 90 per cent of men who are diagnosed can be completely cured if it's detected and treated quickly enough.

Look for:

- a lump or pain in either testicle
- blood-stained ejaculation
- a build-up of fluid inside the scrotum
- a heavy or dragging feeling in the groin or scrotum
- a recent increase in size of either testicle

Information and support for those affected by cancer are available from a number of charities, including: Cancerbackup (telephone freephone 0808 800 1234 (Monday to Friday, 9am to 8pm); www.cancerbackup. org.uk); Cancer Research UK (www.cancerhelp.org.uk); Marie Curie Cancer Care (www.MarieCurie.org.uk); and Macmillan Cancer Support (telephone freephone 0808 808 2020 (Monday to Friday, 9am to 10pm); www.macmillan.org.uk).

Hips and knees

These joints take most of your weight throughout your life and are subjected to huge stresses. Not surprisingly, they are often the first joints to complain of the two great age-linked threats to our lower limbs – arthritis and osteoporosis.

Almost everyone in their fifties and sixties has at least the beginnings of osteoarthritis (so-called 'wear and tear' arthritis) in their hips or knees, or both. This is felt as twinges of pain and stiffness. Hip pain is usually first felt down the front of the thigh, and knee pain either in the joint or in the lower leg. The arthritis attacks and slowly destroys the soft cartilage in the joints that acts like a nylon bearing and is crucial for pain-free movement.

Osteoporosis affects all bones, but often causes problems first in the hips or vertebrae. It's a weakening of the bones caused by 'thinning' or loss of mineral content and it is much more prevalent in women after the menopause. The hips have an angled bracket which attaches the thigh-bone (femur) to the ball-and-socket joint in the pelvis. For this reason, they are particularly vulnerable to fracture caused by osteoporosis.

Maintenance

Arthritis Surprisingly, the best defence against the onset of arthritis is to keep moving. This strengthens your joints as well as your bones and stimulates the repair of worn cartilages. If your arthritis is already quite advanced and painful, you might find that forms of exercise which don't involve bearing your own weight, such as swimming, cycling or pilates, are more comfortable.

Some doctors recommend various dietary supplements to ward off osteoarthritis. The most popular of these are the omega-3 fatty acids obtainable from pharmacies and health food shops, or simply by eating more oily fish (see page 67) or omega-3-boosted margarines.

Osteoporosis Again, the best defence is physical activity, particularly if undertaken earlier in life when bones can be more easily built up and strengthened. Even in our middle years, bones are capable of responding to the demands of exercise, especially if it involves bearing our own weight – walking, running, dancing, tennis, for example. A good healthy balanced diet with plenty of vitamins and minerals is important throughout life for strong, healthy bones. Foods high in calcium and vitamin D (or supplements) may be helpful for people with poorer appetites.

Check-ups

If your hips, knees or other joints are painful, your doctor will probably send you for x-rays in the first instance. You may also need an ultrasound or MRI scan to reveal the state of your joints. Osteoporosis can be assessed by a special type of x-ray called a dexa scan.

Information on arthritis is available from Arthritis Care (telephone helpline 0808 800 4050; www.arthritiscare. org.uk), which provides information and support for people with all types of arthritis throughout the UK. The National

Osteoporosis Society is the only national charity dedicated to improving the prevention, diagnosis and treatment of this fragile bone disease. It offers a wide range of services, including a national helpline and local groups for families and carers (telephone helpline 0845 450 0230 (Monday to Friday, 9am to 5pm); www.nos.org.uk).

Feet

Feet are the most downtrodden part of our body – and yet they are so crucial to our mobility and comfort. And because the circulation in our lower legs and feet is usually the first to feel the effects of age, we shouldn't be surprised if our poor old tootsies start to play up as we attempt to skip nimbly through our middle years. Corns, bunions, fallen arches, hammer toes, fungal nails, whitlows – the list goes on.

Maintenance

Simple routine: careful clipping, frequent bathing, comfortable shoes and time with your feet up.

Check-ups

If you're worried about a foot problem, make an appointment with a NHS or private registered chiropodist or podiatrist.

For further information on foot care, Dr Foot is a commercial website which offers free information and sells a large range of products (telephone 0800 19 53 440; www.drfoot.co.uk). You can find a local registered private chiropodist/podiatrist through Podiatry Pages (www.podiatrypages.co.uk).

Small changes, big difference

There are many other parts of the body that can go wrong in middle age and the bits I've mentioned here can go wrong in lots of other ways. But this isn't meant to be a 'home doctor' book. It's about positive health and keeping everything in good working order.

So let's move into the sunlit uplands of good health. Let's celebrate life.

Feeling good!

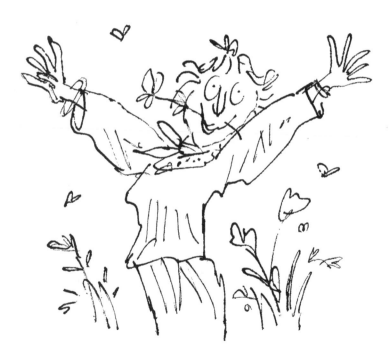

We've come a long way together with this book. We've looked at how being active and eating a balanced diet can boost your health and sense of well-being. We've seen how you can get into shape and shed excess weight. We've tackled the problem of stress and learned how to relax and sleep well. We've looked at threats to health in the form of risky habits, and how to overcome them. And we've gone through a long list of healthchecks to help prevent specific problems that often appear in middle age. That's quite a journey, I know. And you're probably thinking it's all a bit too much. Where would you start?

The answer of course is that you don't have to do the whole lot at once. I've set the elements out in some detail, so you can see the entire strategy. A kind of shop window for a new life. My hope is that you will see something in the window that appeals to you, that you feel you could do, a small change that would make a big difference to your life. Then, maybe, you could find another – and another.

In this way, you can do it. You can make a really big difference to your life through a series of small steps to better health.

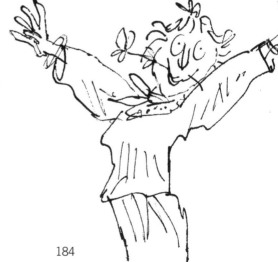

Lucky old us

One good thing about ageing is that it really does creep up on us. It gives us plenty of time to get used to it, although of course we never quite do. First, we notice that policemen and policewomen are looking younger. Then our new doctor doesn't seem quite old enough. And then, within the blink of an eye, we can't help thinking that most prime ministers, presidents and (dreadful thought) even judges are mere striplings.

Another good thing about being older is that it's nowhere near as bad as we thought it was going to be. When we were very young, we thought of people in their fifties and sixties as being ancient, a bit sad, past it, over the hill and far away. But now we are those people, it doesn't seem like that at all. We're still the same youthful us inside. We still have our joys and hopes. We still have lots to see and do and achieve and contribute. Yes, our body is beginning to show its age, our face tells more and more of our life story, and perhaps, at times, we feel quite daunted or downhearted by the unbridled dash of youth sweeping all before it, including us.

Let's just count our blessings. We are the luckiest mid-lifers there have ever been. We baby-boomers have benefited from an unprecedented period of global peace and prosperity. We have lived through a time of incredible advances in medical science. People – in the developed world, at any rate – are living longer and looking younger. Sixty really is the new forty. And commerce and the media are reflecting this fact.

We only have to look around. A whole new marketplace offers us wonderful things to do, wear, participate in, engage with and embrace – all aimed at the over-fifties. There are baby-boomer TV presenters, models, sportspeople, entrepreneurs, decision-makers. There has been a real cultural shift towards a realisation that people of a certain age can be, and often are, the real movers and shakers. And think what we have over the younger generation – wisdom, maturity, self-assuredness, experience, established networks, and the measure of things. Remember all that teenage angst? No, better forget it.

Taking control

I know what you're thinking. You're thinking that this glittering picture of middle age is just a bit too glittering. A bit over-egged. Mid-life through rose-tinted specs. It may be like that for some fortunate people – but it's not like that for you.

But are you quite sure? Or, more specifically, are you quite sure it couldn't be like that for you if you really wanted it to be? My guess is it could – and that's what this book is all about. It's about helping you recognise the difficulties and challenges in maintaining and improving your health and well-being, seeing the benefits of making a few key changes, creating the opportunities to do so, and then just going for it. It's about discovering a virtuous circle: a positive attitude can bring about change, and change can bring about a positive attitude. In short, it's about taking control.

Easier said than done

Yes – life is hard. Yes, there are so many barriers and pitfalls. It's not as though you haven't tried to make changes in the past. But somehow things have conspired against you and, well, who can blame you if you lose heart?

Of course you're absolutely right. It is disappointing to go through the cold turkey of giving up smoking, only to lapse a few weeks or months later. It is demoralising to struggle to lose a few pounds and then see it pile back on again at the mere sight of a Danish pastry. It is depressing to mainline on salads, quaff gallons of juice, handpick the most antioxidant fruits you can find, pump the iron and pound the pavements, only to look in the mirror and still not recognise the disintegrating heap in front of you.

But maybe beauty really is in the eye of the beholder. And maybe the fundamental problem is deep within you. Negative feelings about yourself. A sense of hopelessness. Difficulty in coming to terms with who you are. Letting your looks determine your inner confidence, rather than the other way round. Letting your worries and preoccupations get in the way of everything that's positive about your life.

How on earth can you turn this situation around? Especially if you're struggling to cope with something as all-consuming as an 'empty nest', divorce, retirement, the menopause, a period of illness or the loss of someone very dear to you. Is it surprising that deep down you feel lost and hopeless? It's hard enough just keeping your head above water, let alone striving to be a Superoldie. Can you be blamed for thinking that it's all too much and you might as well throw in the towel and give up on yourself?

Turning the corner

No you can't be blamed. But that's not the point. The point is to try to pick through the wreckage and find signs of life and hope. The point is to realise that you can be rescued from your situation, your circumstances, yourself. Things can change for you. You can change things for you.

How? What's the magic formula?

No magic. It's simple stuff. Say yes, you can do it. Take control. And take one small step at a time. Look again through the pages of this short book. It's crammed with ideas and simple steps you can take. Think about your priorities. What matters most to you? What would be easiest for you to achieve? What could you do that might give you the sense that you're regaining control over your life, and more importantly over your attitude to yourself as a player in your life? It might be something as simple as going for a walk every day or getting your hair done every week. It might be changing to semi-skimmed milk and low-fat cheese, or joining a salsa class. It might be cutting out that lunchtime pint of beer or ringing up that long-lost friend you've been meaning to ring for months (or is it years?). It might be having that check-up you've been putting off, or taking up piano lessons at long last.

Is this really life-changing stuff? Can such small steps really make such a big difference?

Yes, I believe they really can. Not so much each step in itself. But together, as they mount up, they can turn the corner. They can chart the road to a whole new you.

Index

About Age Concern

Age Concern is the UK's largest organisation working for and with older people to enable them to make more of life. We are a federation of over 400 independent charities who share the same name, values and standards and believe that later life should be fulfilling, enjoyable and productive.

Age Concern Books

Age Concern publishes a wide range of bestselling books that help thousands of people each year. They provide practical, trusted advice on subjects ranging from pensions and planning for retirement, to using a computer and surfing the internet. Whether you are caring for someone with a health problem or want to know more about your rights to healthcare, we have something for everyone.

Ordering is easy To order any of our books or request our free catalogue simply choose one of the following options:

☎   **Call us on 0870 44 22 120**

🖰   **Visit our website at www.ageconcern.org.uk/bookshop**

📠   **Email us at sales@ageconcernbooks.co.uk**

You can also buy our books from all good bookshops.

Details of Age Concern head offices in the UK are given below.

Age Concern England
1268 London Road
London SW16 4ER
Tel: 020 8765 7200
www.ageconcern.org.uk

Age Concern Cymru
Ty John Pathy
Units 13 and 14 Neptune Court
Vanguard Way
Cardiff CF24 5PJ
Tel: 029 2043 1555
www.accymru.org.uk

Age Concern Scotland
Causewayside House
160 Causewayside
Edinburgh EH9 1PP
Tel: 0845 833 0200
www.ageconcernscotland.org.uk

Age Concern Northern Ireland
3 Lower Crescent
Belfast BT7 1NR
Tel: 028 9024 5729
www.ageconcernni.org

Free information guides

We have launched a range of comprehensive and **free** information guides designed to answer many of the questions that older people – or those advising them – may have. The guides cover many issues from pensions and benefits to health and education; however *Your health services* and *Healthy living* may be of particular interest to readers of *Feeling Good!*

Order your guides by calling our free information line on **0800 00 99 66** or by downloading them from **www.ageconcern.org.uk/information**

More great books from Age Concern...

Choices in retirement, 4th Edition
Your guide to the essential information

Ro Lyon

Retirement these days means new choices and opportunities. Once you – or your partner – have finally left work, a whole new life awaits you. *Choices in retirement* includes practical information on money issues, working on, housing, health, education and leisure. It's a comprehensive guide for anyone about to retire, as well as for those who've already left work. Whatever dreams, plans and worries you may have, Ro Lyon's friendly and accessible book is here to help you make the very best of the years ahead.

£9.99 • **Paperback** • **978-0-86242-412-1**

How to be a silver surfer, 3rd Edition
A beginner's guide to the internet

Emma Aldridge

'Wonderful ... this book was so easy to understand researching my family tree was a doddle' Tom Hawkins, London

This bestselling guide is perfect for people who are new to the internet and apprehensive about what to do. User-friendly with its clear format, full colour illustrations and simple step-by-step explanations, this guide 'hand-holds' readers through the initial stages of getting to grips with the internet. Learn how to:

- Search the web
- Send an email
- Research your family tree
- Use chat rooms to meet new friends or chat with existing ones
- Take up new hobbies
- Track down the best deals and last-minute bargains

£7.99 • **Paperback** • **978-0-86242-421-3**

Your digital camera made easy
A beginner's guide

Jackie Sherman

This book is the ultimate guide for all beginners starting out with their digital cameras, and those who just want to learn more about how to use one. With its help you'll not only learn how to take great photos, but also how to enhance them using your computer. It explains the following:

- How digital cameras work
- How to choose the right camera
- How to get images onto your computer
- How to edit images and use them creatively
- How to print images, email and store them and lots more

£8.99 • **Paperback** • **978-086242-424-4**

Retiring to Spain
Everything you need to know

Cyril Holbrook

Every year thousands of people dream of retiring abroad. Whether you are looking into your options or planning seriously, this book is a must. It will help to avoid many of the pitfalls, and make the transition to a sunny and healthy retirement a reality. Containing anecdotes and stories to illustrate the points, as well as a list of useful contacts and addresses, this book is the one-stop guide to planning a successful retirement in the sun.

£7.99 • **Paperback** • **978-0-86242-385-8**

Your rights to money benefits 2007/08, 35th Edition
Age Concern's bestselling guide

Sally West

'Essential' *Daily Express*

Now in its 35th edition, *Your Rights 2007-08* gives readers essential up-to-the-minute information on everything they need to know about the full range of state benefits for the over 60s. Using clear, jargon-free language, it reveals a whole host of simple ways to boost finances. This is an indispensable guide, not just for older people, but for their advisers too.

£5.99 • **Paperback** • **978-0-86242-427-5**

Your rights: working after 50
A guide to your employment options

Andrew Harrop & Susie Munro

This is the definitive guide to getting the most out of work after 50 so that you, not other people, decide when you're ready to stop work. Ensure you know your rights in the workplace, learn about support when you're out of work, and find out about the many career opportunities available, from setting up your own business to updating your skills and remaining competitive.

£8.99 • **Paperback** • **978-0-86242-425-1**

Your rights to healthcare, 2nd Edition
Helping older people get the best from the NHS

Lorna Easterbrook

Do you know your way round the NHS? This complete guide explains what NHS services you are entitled to and what to do – and what to expect – when you come into contact with the health service. It provides clear and up-to-date information on areas such as opticians, dentists, GPs, hospitals and support for long-term illness. Although written for older people, the advice offered can benefit anyone using NHS services.

£7.99 • **Paperback** • **978-0-86242-422-0**